DO YOU HAVE THE COMPLETE PICTURE ON HEART HEALTH?

- Have you had your cholesterol levels checked?
- Did the test include your triglyceride levels?
- Do you smoke?
- Do you follow a heart-healthy diet?
- Has your doctor suggested medication to reduce cholesterol and triglyceride levels?

FIND OUT WHAT YOU CAN DO TO REDUCE YOUR RISK OF HEART DISEASE

What You Should Know About TRIGLYCERIDES

The Missing Link in Heart Disease

DENNIS SPRECHER, M.D.

A CMD PUBLISHING BOOK

AN AVON BOOK

WHAT YOU SHOULD KNOW ABOUT TRIGLYCERIDES is not a substitute for sound medical advice. The ideas, procedures, and suggestions in this book are intended to supplement, not replace, the medical advice of a trained medical professional. All matters regarding your health require medical supervision. Consult your physician before adopting the suggestions in this book, as well as about any condition that may require diagnosis or medical attention. The authors and publisher disclaim any liability arising directly or indirectly from the use of this book.

AVON BOOKS, INC.
1350 Avenue of the Americas
New York, New York 10019

Copyright © 2000 by CMD Publishing, a division of Current Medical Directions, Inc.
Illustration by Philip Ashley, C.M.I.
Published by arrangement with CMD Publishing, a division of Current Medical Directions, Inc.
Library of Congress Catalog Card Number: 99-94990
ISBN: 0-380-80940-0
www.avonbooks.com/wholecare

First WholeCare Printing: January 2000

WHOLECARE TRADEMARK REG. U.S. PAT. OFF. AND IN OTHER COUNTRIES, MARCA REGISTRADA, HECHO EN U.S.A.

Printed in the U.S.A.

WCD   10 9 8 7 6 5 4 3 2 1

Contents

What You Should Know About TRIGLYCERIDES

How the Heart Works

John, age 27, is a graduate student at the local university. When I first met John he was burning the candle at both ends. In addition to taking classes, he was teaching writing courses to undergraduates and working nights to put himself through school. He came to my office complaining of heart palpitations that were making it difficult for him to fall asleep at night. His concern that something might be wrong with his heart was adding to his anxiety. John's medical history revealed that he had been diagnosed with a mild case of mitral valve prolapse, a relatively common congenital (present at birth) heart defect that strikes about 5% to 7% of Americans. In this disorder, the one-way valve between the two chambers on the left side of the heart fails to close completely, allowing a small quantity of blood to flow backward in the wrong direction. After conducting a physical exam and checking John's blood pressure, I ordered an electrocardiogram and some other tests to better evaluate how his heart was beating. John was relieved to hear that the organ was functioning well and that he was in fine cardiovascular health. I explained that people with his type of heart murmur sometimes complain of heart palpitations or anxiety when they are under stress. The six cups of coffee a day John was drinking may also have been a contributing factor. I was pleased to hear that John was already trying some nondrug therapies such as meditation to help him relax. I told him that using techniques to alleviate or manage stress may also help to reduce his risk of developing cardiovascular disease.

For most of recorded history, the heart was considered the seat of the soul and the source of human intellect. Even our cave-dwelling ancestors apparently attributed some mystical significance to the organ. While we can only speculate as to what the heart represented to them, we can still see their portrayals of it in renderings of animals they left behind in the dark recesses of European caves. Most writers and thinkers throughout the ages, suspecting the heart's importance if not its true significance, believed that our most passionate emotions and refined thoughts sprang from the steady beating beneath our breast. This cultural history of the heart as a symbol of love and devotion is not so easy to cast off. We still "cross our hearts," exchange heart-shaped cards and candies on Valentine's Day, and instinctively place a hand over our breast when emotions overwhelm us. Today we know that our knowledge of the world around us and our emotional reaction to it have a lot more to do with our heads than our hearts. Yet now that we have a greater understanding of what the heart is and how it actually works, we are no less fascinated by it.

Q: What is the heart?
A: In the simplest terms, the heart is a powerful pump that helps to circulate blood to all the organs and tissues in your body. The heart begins beating a few weeks after conception and continues to beat ceaselessly for a lifetime, averaging about 70 beats a minute in adults (100,000 beats a day). The blood it pumps delivers oxygen and essential nutrients to every part of your body, from your head to your toes. In addition to transporting oxygen and food, blood also performs clean-up duties. It removes waste products such as carbon dioxide from your tissues and carries them to the lungs or other organs to be filtered and expelled. The heart is the "prime mover" of your circulatory system—the system composed mainly of the heart, lungs, and blood vessels (flexible tubes that carry blood through the body). With the help of the heart, the 10 pints (a little over a gallon) of blood contained in an average adult complete the round trip from the heart to the far reaches of the body and back again about 1,600 times each day—roughly once every minute. The heart beats over *2.5 billion times* during a seventy-year life span!

Q: How big is the heart?
A: Your heart is about the same size as your fist (unless you have unusually large or small hands). This is true for men and women, adults and children alike. Contrary to what some women may suspect, men generally have larger hearts than the female sex—literally speaking, at least. The average male heart weighs about 10 ounces—a

woman's heart usually weighs a few ounces less. If you are like most people, you probably place your hand over the left side of your chest to indicate the location of your heart. This is mainly a symbolic gesture enforced by custom. The heart actually resides approximately in the center of the chest, between the lungs. Lying beneath the sternum (breastbone) and above the diaphragm (a fanlike muscle lying between the chest and abdominal cavities), the heart is one of the most well-protected organs in the body. The shape of the heart is a little more difficult to visualize. It has been described in a variety of ways, from an upside-down pear to a paper cup. Roughly speaking, the heart resembles the shape of a blunt cone, with the widest part being at the top. It sits in the chest cavity at an angle. The lower, more narrow end of the heart points to the left side of the chest and sticks out a little from underneath the sternum. Because that part of the heart contains a powerful pumping chamber and is located nearest to the surface of the chest, most people mistakenly assume that the heart is located on the left side.

Q: What do the inside and outside of the heart look like?
A: Probably not what you expect. First of all, the heart is not one pump but two. These two pumping mechanisms are located side by side within the muscular shell of the heart. Though not identical, they are very similar in terms of how they work. The powerful pump on the left side of the heart is responsible for circulating blood throughout the body. The less powerful pumping chamber on the right forces blood into the lungs and then back to the heart. These two pumps must work in harmony to keep your blood circulating properly. They are separated from each other by a wall of muscle called the septum. *Wall* is the key word here. When the heart is working properly,

blood does not cross from one side of the heart to the other. There is a good reason for this. Though the heart is a single organ, the blood that passes through each side of the heart is *not* the same. Blood that enters the right side of the heart is "old" blood that has just returned from another round trip through the body. It has unloaded its cargo of oxygen and other nutrients during its journey and is now heavy with carbon dioxide waste. It has even changed color, having taken on a deep blue or purplish hue. This blood needs to be recycled in the lungs, where it receives fresh oxygen, before it can be used to serve the needs of the body. So what about the blood in the other side of the heart? The blood entering the left side of the heart is newly oxygenated blood that has come straight from the lungs. It is bright red in color and ready to make its trip through the circulatory system. By separating one side of the heart from the other, the septum prevents old blood from mixing with the new. The outer portion of the heart is primarily a layer of cardiac muscle called the myocardium. The heart itself is enclosed in a thin, translucent sac called the pericardium. This deceptively delicate membrane helps to protect the heart from being invaded by infections from other parts of the body such as the lungs.

◆
Circulation: The Paths Your Blood Takes

We often refer to "circulation" as if it were a single system. It is actually three separate processes that work together as a whole to ensure that blood reaches every part of the body and is recycled with fresh oxygen on a regular basis. All three of your body's circulatory systems, which you can think of as loops or circuits of blood-carrying vessels, start and end with the heart. Blood flows through all these systems at the same time, your blood vessels are never empty.

- *Body.* This is the largest system. Fresh, oxygenated blood is pumped by the heart through an extensive network of blood vessels that reaches into every corner of your body. Blood then returns to the heart. This process is called systemic (whole-body) circulation.
- *Lungs.* Once blood has made its circuit through the body, it returns to the heart via the right side. This bluish, deoxygenated blood is then pumped through the nearby lungs to unload carbon dioxide and pick up a fresh supply of oxygen. Blood then returns to the left side of the heart. This loop, from the heart to the lungs and back to the heart, is referred to as pulmonary circulation.
- *Heart.* You can think of this system, which allows the heart to nourish itself, as an important detour. During systemic circulation, a portion of the life-sustaining blood pumped by the heart is sent right back to the organ, which needs oxygen and nutrients no less than other parts of the body. This process is called coronary circulation.

◆

Q: How do the pumps inside the heart work?
A: The pump on the left side of the heart is the more powerful of the two. It has to be, because its job is to push blood through the vast network of blood vessels that reaches into every corner of your body. This side of the heart is composed of two chambers, one sitting atop the other. The cavity on top is called the left atrium. It is a filling chamber that receives blood that has just come

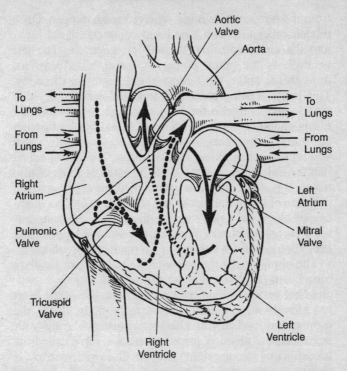

Blood flow through the heart. Deoxygenated blood that has made its circuit through the body enters the right atrium of the heart and then flows through the right ventricle. The blood passes into the lungs, where it receives fresh oxygen. The freshly oxygenated blood enters the left atrium of the heart and then flows into the left ventricle. Blood then passes into the aorta and its branches, which brings blood into every corner of the body. Both of these circuits of blood flow through the heart simultaneously and continuously.

from the lungs, where it has received fresh oxygen. Once this chamber fills with blood and contracts, blood flows into the chamber below it—the left ventricle. The left ventricle is the pump proper. It forces blood outward through the aorta, the largest blood vessel in the body. This is the starting point for the round-trip journey that blood makes through the body. In order to get from the filling chamber to the pump itself, blood passes through the mitral valve. This is not similar to the sort of valve you replace when fixing a leaky faucet. The mitral valve, like the other valves of the heart, is made of folds of thin tissue. It is a one-way valve that opens in response to the pressure of the blood that passes through it. Once a quantity of blood has gone through the mitral valve, its billowy layers fold back upon themselves, overlapping and keeping blood from flowing in the opposite direction.

The pump on the right side of the heart is practically a mirror image of the one on the left. It also is a two-chamber system. Blood entering the right side of the heart has already made a circuit through the body. It fills the right atrium. When this chamber squeezes during your heartbeat, the blood is forced through a valve called the tricuspid and into the right ventricle. The right ventricle is similar to the pumping chamber on the left side. The right pump is less strong because its job is to push old blood into the nearby lungs where it can be reoxygenated. The familiar *thump-thump* sound of your heartbeat corresponds to the dual-pumping action of the heart—the contractions of its chambers and closing of the valves.

A Look Inside the Heart

The heart is made up of four chambers that contract in a coordinated way to push blood through the interior of the organ and to other parts of the body. The heart also contains four valves that help to regulate the passage of blood.

The Left Side of the Heart

- *Left atrium.* This is the filling chamber above the left ventricle. Blood entering the left side of the heart fills this cavity before passing into the pump below.
- *Left ventricle.* The more powerful of the two pumps, the left ventricle forces newly oxygenated, bright red blood out of the heart and into all the tissues and organs of the body.
- *Mitral valve.* The mitral valve is the passage between the left atrium and the pump below.
- *Aortic valve.* Blood leaving the left side of the heart must pass through this valve in order to enter the aorta, the heart's main exit tube.

The Right Side of the Heart

- *Right atrium.* This is the filling chamber that sits atop the right ventricle.
- *Right ventricle.* The right ventricle is the low-pressure pump that propels old, deoxygenated blood along its short circuit through the lungs (where it receives fresh oxygen) and back to the heart, which it now enters on the left side. This pump is weaker than the pump on the left side.
- *Tricuspid valve.* This valve connects the right atrium to the right ventricle.
- *Pulmonic valve.* This valve regulates blood flowing from the right side of the heart into the artery leading to the lungs.

Q: What makes the heart beat?

A: Every heartbeat begins with a spark—literally a small electrical charge. This current originates in the sinus node, an area of tissue in the right filling chamber. (The sinus node is sometimes referred to as a natural pace-maker.) The current sweeps across your heart and triggers the coordinated squeezing of the chambers—what you perceive as your heart beating. These electrical impulses are the spark of life in a very real sense. In their absence, the heart and circulatory system come to an abrupt halt. When the current stops, you stop.

Q: How does blood get from place to place in the body?

A: Blood gets from one place to another by traveling through a vast network of blood vessels. Blood vessels are flexible tubes designed to carry blood in one direction only. They come in different types and sizes that reflect their different jobs. There are three main kinds: Arteries, veins, and capillaries. Once blood leaves the left side of the heart, it travels *away* from the organ through arteries. Veins are the means by which blood makes its way *back* to the heart. Arteries and veins generally run side by side throughout your body, like parallel highways moving in opposite directions. Capillaries are the tiny vessels that connect arteries with veins. It is in the capillaries that blood delivers oxygen and food to nearby tissue and takes on carbon dioxide. This network of blood vessels is *very* extensive. How extensive, you wonder? Consider this: If you removed all the blood vessels from an adult and laid them end to end, they would stretch for about 60,000 miles!

Q: What happens when blood is pumped out of the left side of the heart?

A: Blood that leaves the left side of the heart for other parts of the body does so via the aorta. As you saw earlier in the chapter, blood traveling away from the heart is newly oxygenated and bright red in color. The trip starts when blood is pumped out of the powerful left ventricle. Once blood enters the aorta, it branches into smaller and smaller arteries as it gets further away from the heart. Healthy arteries are elastic and composed of several layers of tissue. The middle layer is actually made of muscle. With each heartbeat, blood courses through your arteries, which swell to accommodate the flow of blood and then snap back slightly. The tensing and relaxing of muscles during everyday activity gives blood flow a "push," helping to propel the blood forward along its journey. Any disease that causes arteries to become weaker or less elastic can damage the circulatory system and threaten your health. As you might expect, the inside of a healthy artery is very smooth, encouraging the flow of blood.

Q: After flowing through the arteries, where does this blood go?

A: Eventually blood reaches the capillaries. These are the smallest blood vessels and they reach into all the tissues and organs of your body. In a way, capillaries are the destination of blood that is pumped out of the left side of the heart. It is here that red blood cells deliver their life-sustaining cargo of oxygen and nutrients while absorbing the carbon dioxide (the waste product of the body's metabolic processes) that needs a trip to the lungs. This process is one of the most interesting aspects of the circulatory system. It is difficult for most people to appreciate just how narrow the capillaries are or how thin are their walls. When blood moves through a capillary, it is a very tight squeeze. These vessels are so narrow that red blood cells must line up single file in order to keep moving! The walls of these vessels are also remarkably thin—in fact, they are just one cell thick. They are so thin that gases like oxygen and carbon dioxide simply pass *through* the walls of the capillaries. Oxygen is released by red blood cells into the adjoining tissue while carbon dioxide crosses over and takes the place of the newly departed oxygen.

Q: How does blood get back to the heart?

A: Once blood has passed through the capillaries—releasing its oxygen payload and picking up carbon dioxide—it makes its way back to the heart via the veins. Veins are the one-way highways that lead *back* to the heart. They carry the dark-blue blood heavy with waste products like carbon dioxide. They run alongside the arteries and have a similar structure. Veins also have an elastic, muscular middle layer, but it is weaker than that of the arteries. Veins do not need to be as strong because the blood making its way back to the heart is under less pressure. Veins have also evolved a feature that arteries lack—they have one-way valves resembling those of the heart. These valves are designed to keep blood from flowing in the wrong direction. The journey that blood takes back to the heart is often in an upward direction, against the force of gravity. When you consider the long, upward trek that blood must take from the tips of your toes all the way back to your heart, it is easy to see why nature employed valves as a safeguard against backward flow. Once blood reaches the heart, it enters the right side via two large veins called the vena cava (the "heart's veins"). While deep veins transport most blood back to the heart, some veins are visible just under your skin. Take a look at your hands or arms. Do you see a few bluish vessels showing through? This is your blood making a return trip all the way back up to your heart.

Q: At what point does blood get recycled in the lungs?

A: Once blood has made the round trip through your body, it comes back to its starting point, the heart, entering the atrium on the right side. This blood is dark blue or purple in color because its red blood cells are now carrying carbon dioxide instead of oxygen. After filling the atrium, this old blood is pushed into the low-pressure ventricle below and pumped out of the right side of the heart and into the nearby lungs. It is in the lungs that blood unloads its cargo of carbon dioxide and picks up oxygen. Let us take a look at how the effortless act of breathing supplies oxygen to your blood and at the same time expels waste gases rounded up by your blood on its trip through the body.

- *Breathing in.* When you inhale, the muscles of your diaphragm contract, drawing oxygen through a number of passages in order to reach the lungs. It enters the larynx (voice box) and proceeds through the trachea (windpipe) into the chest cavity. There the trachea splits into the two main breathing tubes, called the bronchi, which continue to divide into numerous passages called the bronchial tubes. These tubes get more and more narrow as they reach deep into the tissue of your lungs. At the tips of these bronchial tubes are millions of tiny, balloonlike sacs called alveoli. Once oxygen reaches the alveoli, it is ready to make the short hop from these sacs into the blood that is flowing through a web of nearby capillaries. In the rest of the body, red blood cells trade their oxygen for carbon dioxide. In the lungs, the process is reversed. Here these cells release carbon dioxide and attract the oxygen molecules contained in the alveoli.

- *Breathing out.* Once the exchange is made, your diaphragm muscles relax and the carbon dioxide that has crossed from your capillaries into the alveoli is now forced out of the body via the same route that oxygen took to reach the lungs. Meanwhile the newly oxygenated blood makes it way back to the heart, completing the cycle of pulmonary circulation.

Q: What about the heart itself? Doesn't it need food and fuel just like any other part of the body?

A: That is an excellent question. After all, the heart pumps blood to all areas of the body to ensure that they get the oxygen and nutrients they need. But while it is doing this, who provides nourishment for the heart—an organ with the same needs as other vital organs? The answer: Nature devised a way that the heart could feed itself. Once blood leaves the left side of the heart via the aorta, some of that blood immediately enters the coronary arteries. These are the arteries that serve the heart. They get smaller as they wind their way around the outer surface of the heart muscle. Eventually they branch off into capillaries, where the exchange of oxygen and carbon dioxide takes place. Due to its location, the heart is actually the first organ to receive and be nourished by the very blood that it itself is pumping out! If the heart did not receive oxygen and other nutrients, it would not be able to perform its job.

Q: What is blood?
A: Blood is the fluid that sustains life. The sophisticated apparatus of your circulatory system would grind to a halt without it. Much of your blood is a watery base called plasma. This plasma conveys a variety of other substances and gases (fats, vitamins, minerals, and oxygen, just to name a few examples), each with different jobs and destinations within the body. Some of these substances—red blood cells, for example—are permanent ingredients of blood, while others may enter and then exit the bloodstream. For this reason, the chemical composition of your blood is constantly changing, from day to day and from hour to hour. So when we refer to the term *blood* we mean two things: Blood is a *medium* that carries other substances from place to place in the body. It is also the *sum total* of your blood's ingredients at a particular moment.

Blood and its components perform many functions. Blood delivers oxygen and nutrients to your organs and tissues. Most of these nutrients are derived from what you eat and drink. Blood also retrieves wastes in gas and liquid form and drops them off in the lungs or kidneys where they are excreted. Hormones are carried along the bloodstream on their way to and from various organs and glands, delivering the chemical messages that help to regulate important processes in the body. Disease-fighting white blood cells also prowl the circulatory system in search of harmful invaders. Some important aspects of blood are described below. See Chapter 5 for more information about triglycerides and your blood.

- *Plasma.* Roughly half your blood is plasma. This clear, yellowish liquid is made mostly of water. You can think of plasma as the river or current that transports most of the other substances in your blood. Plasma is not the same thing as serum, which is also part of blood. Serum describes the fluid that remains after platelets and other clotting agents are removed from plasma.

• **Red blood cells.** These cells do most of the heavy lifting in the bloodstream, alternately hauling oxygen or carbon dioxide. Their double duty is to deliver oxygen to your tissues via the capillaries and pick up the refuse left over by your body's metabolism. Carbon dioxide waste is hauled back to the heart and eventually the lungs, where it is dropped off for expulsion. A protein in red blood cells called hemoglobin is what gives blood its red color. Hemoglobin contains the element iron, which is like a magnet for oxygen and carbon dioxide alike. Red blood cells are able to carry oxygen or carbon dioxide because these gases bond with the hemoglobin inside. One drop of blood contains millions of red blood cells. They live about four months and are constantly replaced by new red blood cells produced in your bones.

• **White blood cells.** White blood cells are the warriors of your bloodstream. Traveling alongside the cargo-carrying red blood cells, they are constantly patrolling your body for trouble in the form of disease-causing microorganisms. A drop of blood contains roughly 10,000 to 20,000 white blood cells. This number is basically a "maintenance" force. If white blood cells have trouble containing a threat to your health, the number of these cells can increase as the call goes out for reinforcements. White blood cells live only for days or weeks and are replaced by new cells of the same type.

Q: What is blood pressure?

A: Blood pressure is the force that blood exerts on the walls of the vessels. At one time or another most of us have felt conscious of the blood coursing through our bodies—perhaps in times of stress or after a vigorous workout at the gym. These are the moments when we are most aware that our blood is literally under pressure. While it is true that substances in your blood are constantly entering and exiting the stream, for the most part your blood is contained in the closed circuits of your blood vessel systems. Blood pressure is not the same in all parts of your body. For example, blood making the return trip via veins is under less pressure than the blood traveling through arteries.

When doctors measure blood pressure they are measuring the pressure of the blood in your arteries. Ever wonder why your blood pressure measurement is always in the form of two numbers? This is because doctors measure blood pressure during the two main phases of your heartbeat—the systolic (beating) and diastolic (resting) phases. Systolic blood pressure, the first number given by your doctor, is the pressure of blood in your arteries when your heart muscles are contracting during a heartbeat. Diastolic pressure, the second number, is the pressure of your blood when your heart is momentarily resting between beats. As most of us know, blood pressure does not remain constant. It is normal for it to climb during physical exertion and dip when you are sleeping. Anxiety can boost pressure as well. It has even become popular to refer to our stress levels in terms of our blood pressure: "This job is driving my blood pressure through the roof!" But while it is natural for blood pressure to go up and down over the course of a day, pressure that stays consistently high can put too much strain on the cardiovascular system and damage blood vessels. As you will see in Chapter 3, hypertension (high blood pressure) can contribute to heart attack and stroke.

Blood Pressure: How High Is Too High?

A healthy blood pressure level can vary from person to person. Normal pressure for the systolic phase is below 140 mm Hg. During the diastolic phase, a normal reading is under 90 mm Hg. The ranges listed below apply to adults.

Category	Systolic (mm Hg)	Diastolic (mm Hg)
Optimal	120	80
Normal	<130	<85
High normal	130–139	85–89
Hypertension	≥ 140	≥ 90

Source: The Sixth Report of the Joint National Committee on Prevention, Detection, Evaluation, and Treatment of High Blood Pressure. Bethesda, MD: National Institutes of Health, National Heart, Lung, and Blood Institute, 1997.

What Is Cardiovascular Disease?

Eddie, age 63, is a truck driver with an independent streak and his own rig. Eddie never paid much attention to his heart health or to warnings by friends and family to lose weight or trim the fat from his diet. Long hours on the road meant that he got little exercise and relied on the greasy fare offered by roadside burger joints and truck stops. Eddie experienced a rude awakening several years ago when he suffered a heart attack and had to undergo coronary artery bypass surgery. This is a procedure that improves blood flow to the heart by removing a blood vessel from another part of the body and using it to bypass a severely clogged coronary artery. Eddie viewed his recovery as a second chance and wisely decided to make his cardiovascular health a priority in his life. He now gets aerobic exercise at least three times a week—he

*makes time even if he is on the road—and carefully fol-
lows the dietary regimen he crafted with a registered
dietician.*

Progress has taken its toll on the American heart. Many
of the modern-day technological advances that we like to
believe are making our lives easier are actually putting a
heavy burden on our hearts and blood vessels (flexible
tubes that carry blood through the body). The way we
work and eat have changed considerably over the last
century or so. For one thing, we no longer need to expend
much physical energy to earn our daily bread. In our
great-grandparents' time, when heart disease was not the
killer that it is today, work was synonymous with manual
labor and meals were typically homemade. Today
mechanical beasts of burden do much of the labor that
once required the sweat of our brow—from bulldozers to
electric kitchen mixers. Planes, trains, and automobiles
spare us the trouble of traveling by foot, and factories
mass-produce most of the food we eat—food that we say
we are too busy to prepare ourselves. The rich, high-fat
foods that have become staples of our nation's diet—
from hamburgers and hot dogs to the cakes and candies in
your local convenience store—were only occasional
indulgences in the not-so-distant past. America's cardiovascular health suffered as a result of our sedentary habits
and a growing reliance on mass-produced, processed
foods. Heart disease became the world's most serious
epidemic.

Now America is starting to fight back in the war
against heart disease. Some of our gains have been
impressive. In the decade ending in 1995, the death rate
due to heart attack dropped almost 30%. We are recognizing that, in a world of desk-bound jobs and fast-food
joints, it often takes an extra effort to keep our hearts and
blood vessels in tip-top condition. We can best accom-

plish this by sticking to a "heart smart" diet and getting regular exercise. As a nation we still have some distance to cover. Though largely preventable, cardiovascular disease remains the number one killer of American men and women, claiming over a million lives each year. Roughly half these deaths are due to heart attacks. Almost 70 million people in this country suffer from some form of cardiovascular disease, usually in the form of hypertension (high blood pressure) or coronary artery disease (CAD). You may be surprised to learn that nearly as many people die from cardiovascular disease as from all other causes *combined,* including accidents and cancer. This equal opportunity killer does not discriminate, striking men and women alike and people of all races. (Although men tend to develop heart problems at a younger age, women suffer from these diseases at the same rate a decade or so after menopause.) In this chapter we focus on some of the most important types of cardiovascular disease, including those that can lead to heart attack and stroke. See Chapter 3 for information on how to evaluate your risk factors and prevent cardiovascular disease.

Q: What is cardiovascular disease?

A: This term is used to describe any of a number of disorders that affect the circulatory system. This system is composed mainly of the heart and blood vessels and is responsible for providing oxygen and nutrients to the tissues and organs throughout your body. Cardiovascular disease includes clogged coronary arteries (the three arteries that supply the heart with oxygen) as well as diseases affecting arteries and veins in other parts of the body. Hypertension is also a form of cardiovascular disease, as are disorders that originate in the heart or its valves. These problems can be congenital (present at birth) or due to an injury or infection. Most heart and blood vessel diseases develop over a period of years as arteries that supply the heart or brain with blood slowly become clogged from a buildup of fat and other substances. These obstructions in your circulatory system can choke the passages that nourish your heart and brain with oxygen-laden blood. The result may be a heart attack or stroke. It is important to understand the relationship between different components of your circulatory system. Chapter 1 explains how this system works as a unit and how one part often depends on another to function properly. Clogged blood vessels, for example, can increase your risk of hypertension and stroke, while hypertension itself can damage blood vessels and increase the likelihood of heart attack.

Q: What is CAD?
A: We should back up a bit. As you saw in Chapter 1, the coronary arteries are the three vessels that wind their way around the heart. These small arteries nourish the heart with oxygen-rich blood pumped out of the nearby aorta near the top of the heart. Coronary arteries (which differ in size depending on gender) get smaller as they carry blood away from the aorta and into the heart muscle itself by way of capillaries. Healthy coronary arteries are smooth and slippery on the inside, allowing a sufficient quantity of blood to flow through them and into the tissue of the heart. In the almost 14 million Americans who live with CAD, the type of heart disease associated with heart attack, one or more of these arteries becomes clogged or obstructed due to the buildup of plaque. This is not the sort of plaque that accumulates on teeth. Plaques that form in arteries are composed of a number of substances, including cholesterol (a fatty substance found in certain foods and also manufactured by the body), the mineral calcium, fibrin (a substance that helps blood to clot), and cellular debris. Atherosclerosis is the process by which

arteries become thickened and hardened due to plaque buildup. It is tempting to describe plaques as garbage heaps deposited on the walls of arteries, and there is some truth in this metaphor. But it is also important to understand that most of the ingredients of plaque are necessary for good health. Cholesterol, for example, is necessary for the formation of cell membranes and the production of hormones (chemical message carriers). Calcium helps to build strong bones among its other important functions.

It is when these substances accumulate on the walls of arteries that they present a problem. This is because they do not *belong* there. Arteries are your body's main thoroughfares for blood leaving the heart. Plaques, which often begin to develop during childhood and may continue to grow for decades, are hard deposits that thicken the wall of an artery, forcing blood to squeeze through a narrower than normal space. Watching blood squeeze through a clogged artery is a little like watching rush-hour traffic merge from several lanes of highway into one. The result? Blood flow to the heart—the "prime mover" of your circulatory system—is reduced and the organ does not pump as efficiently. If CAD progresses, life-threatening obstructions may form at the site of plaque buildup. These are like roadblocks that completely block the flow of blood to part of the heart—what we refer to as a heart attack. These total blockages can occur one of two ways. Often the plaque in a coronary artery ruptures and a blood clot (called a thrombus) forms, completely obstructing that particular route to the heart.

Q: What are the symptoms of coronary artery disease?
A: Often none. Angina, which is chronic chest pain triggered by physical or emotional strain and relieved by rest,

may be the only obvious indication of clogged arteries. Many people with CAD experience fatal heart attacks before realizing that they have clogged arteries.

Q: How is it treated?
A: Long-term diet and lifestyle changes are the main features of treatment. Medications such as nitroglycerin, beta blockers, and calcium channel blockers may be used to dilate (widen) the affected arteries, help reduce the strain on the heart, and relieve the pain associated with angina. Less often, surgical procedures such as balloon dilation or coronary bypass grafting may be necessary to clear blockages.

◆

Collateral Circulation: A Natural Detour around Clogged Arteries?

What if your body was able to reroute blood around plaque deposits in your coronary arteries? Collateral blood vessels are your body's attempt to do just this. Everybody has these "reserve" blood vessels, but in most of us they remain in microscopic form and do not serve any real purpose. However, collateral blood vessels undergo a fascinating change in certain people with CAD—they enlarge and become operational. Sometimes they act as bridges between one coronary artery and another. If the former artery is obstructed due to plaque buildup, collateral blood vessels can divert some of the blood from the narrowed artery into a nearby and less constricted one. These reserve blood vessels can also allow blood flow to bypass plaque in an artery by detouring it *around* the site of the plaque. In these cases, collateral blood vessels actually connect one section of an artery with another section further down the line: Think of the way cars are sometimes waved onto the shoulder of the road to avoid an accident scene and then allowed to enter the main highway again once the obstruction is behind them. Collateral blood vessels essentially provide an alternate route for blood trying to reach the heart. So why are these blood vessel detours activated in some people with CAD but not in others? Doctors suspect that genetics play a strong role, but the process may also have to do with the speed with which the artery has become blocked; if the blockage occurred very quickly, collateral blood vessels would not have had enough time to have developed.

◆

Q: What is a heart attack and how is it different from CAD?
A: CAD is the result of stenosis, or narrowing, of a coronary artery. Clogged coronary arteries slowly reduce the blood supply to the heart; if the blockage is extreme, the blood flow can be reduced to only a trickle. A heart attack is a cardiac *event* that occurs when the blood supply to part of the heart muscle is not just slowed but actually stopped (or severely reduced). This can happen when one of the coronary arteries that supplies blood to the heart is blocked by an obstruction—usually a blood clot that forms near a rupture of atherosclerotic plaque. When blood supply is cut off from an area of the heart muscle, the affected cells

become damaged or actually die because they are starved of oxygen. Human death or disability can result depending on which part of the heart is affected, how much heart muscle is damaged, and how quickly medical attention is sought. About half the people who suffer fatal heart attacks each year die within one hour of experiencing the first symptoms. Heart attacks can also be triggered by involuntary muscle contractions of a coronary artery. When this happens, the artery narrows and blood flow to part of the heart muscle sharply decreases or stops. These spasms of coronary arteries can occur in healthy vessels and clogged arteries alike. Exactly what causes them is unclear. See the section on variant angina later in this chapter for more information on coronary artery spasm.

◆

Warning Signs of a Heart Attack

Recognizing the warning signs of a heart attack is often the key to survival. They are not as obvious as you might think. The sensation may range from pressure or tightness to a crushing pain in the chest. This pain can radiate down the arm or spread to the shoulders, neck, and head. These feelings of pain or pressure may continue for several hours. According to the American Heart Association (AHA), the warnings signs of a heart attack include:

- Uncomfortable pressure, fullness, squeezing, or pain in the center of the chest lasting more than a few minutes
- Pain spreading to the shoulders, neck, or arms

• Chest discomfort with lightheadedness, fainting, sweating, nausea, or shortness of breath

Source: Reproduced with permission. American Heart Association World Wide Web site http://www.americanheart. org/warning.html. Copyright American Heart Association.

◆

Q: What can I do if I think I am having a heart attack?
A: That is a great question. The fact is that most heart attacks can be survived if quick action is taken. During a heart attack, one or more of the arteries feeding the heart becomes totally obstructed. The affected heart muscle begins to die about 20 minutes after the blood supply is interrupted, so it is important to recognize that the "clock is ticking" and respond without delay. Simply *knowing* the warning signs of a heart attack is a crucial first step. Most people who have heart attacks experience some degree of chest pain but others feel only a squeezing sensation or heaviness in the chest. Women who suffer heart attacks tend to describe the pain as diffuse while men usually report that their pain is sharper and confined to a smaller region of the chest. Some people—particularly those over age 70, those with diabetes, and those who have had heart attacks in the past—have "silent" heart attacks that are not preceded by chest pain or pressure. In these cases, being short of breath or having an upset stomach may be the only indications that an attack has begun. If you think you are experiencing a heart attack, the first step is to seek emergency help by dialing 911 and requesting an ambulance. You should never attempt to drive yourself to the hospital once an attack has begun because you

may lose consciousness while en route. It is wiser to wait for the emergency services team, which can begin treating you on the scene and in the ambulance on the way to the emergency room. Sit or lie down while you wait for help to arrive and do not exert yourself.

If your doctor has prescribed nitroglycerin tablets for you, place one tablet under your tongue as soon as you begin to experience symptoms of a heart attack. This medication dilates the coronary arteries and allows more blood to reach the heart. You may take a *total* of three doses spaced five minutes apart while waiting for the ambulance to arrive. You should take nitroglycerin only if your doctor has prescribed it for you—it can be fatal in people with certain kinds of heart disease. You should also take an *uncoated* aspirin in addition to the nitroglycerin. If your doctor has not prescribed nitroglycerin for you, take an uncoated aspirin—even if you are not certain that you are having an attack. Aspirin helps to thin the blood and may increase blood flow to the heart during the critical early stages of a heart attack. If your heart stops during the attack (cardiac arrest) and the ambulance team has not yet arrived, cardiopulmonary resuscitation (CPR) can be a life saver—assuming that there is someone on the spot who knows how to administer it. CPR helps to ensure that oxygen-laded blood is reaching some parts of the body while the heart is temporarily shut down. If any of your family members or close friends have heart disease, contact your local hospital about learning CPR. If you know CPR you may be able to help revive a loved one who suffers cardiac arrest during a heart attack.

◆

Performing CPR

When attempting to perform CPR, remember the ABCs—airway, breathing, and circulation. The following instructions, provided by AHA, explain how to perform CPR on adults or children over age eight.

Assessment

Find out if the person who has collapsed is responsive by gently shaking a shoulder and shouting, "Are you all right?" If the person does not respond, shout for help. If a helper is available, send that person to call emergency medical services (911 or other local number). If no one on the scene offers to help, make the 911 call yourself.

A—Airway

To open the airway, gently lift the chin with one hand while pushing down on the forehead with your other hand. You want to tilt the head back. Once the airway is open, lean over and put your ear close to the victim's mouth.

- Look at the chest for movement.
- Listen for the sound of breathing.
- Feel for breath on your cheek.

If the victim is breathing, roll the person onto his or her side (the recovery position). If none of the above signs is present, the person is not breathing. If opening the airway does not cause the person to spontaneously start breathing, you will have to provide rescue breathing.

B—Breathing

The best way to give rescue breathing is by using the mouth-to-mouth technique. Using the thumb and forefinger of your hand (which is on the person's forehead), pinch the person's nose shut. Be sure to keep the heel of your hand in place so the person's head remains tilted. Keep your other hand under the person's chin, lifting up. As you keep an air-tight seal with your mouth on the victim's mouth, immediately give two full breaths.*

C—Circulation

After giving two full breaths, find the person's carotid artery pulse to see if the heart is still beating. To find the carotid artery pulse, take your hand that is lifting the chin and find the person's Adam's apple. Slide the tips of your fingers down the groove beside the Adam's apple and feel for the pulse. If you cannot find the pulse, besides providing rescue breathing, you will have to provide artificial circulation by external chest compression (see below).

External Chest Compression

External chest compressions provide artificial blood circulation. When you apply rhythmic pressure on the lower half of the victim's breastbone, you force the heart to pump blood. To do external chest compression properly, kneel beside the victim's chest. With the middle and index fingers of your hand nearest the person's legs, find the notch where the bottom rims of the two halves of the rib cage meet in the middle of the chest. Now put the heel of one hand on the sternum (breastbone) next to the fingers that found the notch. Put your other hand on top of the hand that is in position. Be sure to keep your fingers up off the chest wall. It may be easier to do this if you interlock your fingers.

Bring your shoulders directly over the victim's sternum and press down, keeping your arms straight. If the victim is an adult, depress the sternum about 1½ to 2 inches. Then completely relax the pressure on the sternum. Do not remove your hands from the victim's sternum, but do let the chest rise to its normal position between compressions. Relaxation and compression should take equal amounts of time.

If you must give both rescue breathing and external chest compressions, the proper rate is 15 chest compressions to two breaths. You must compress at a rate of 80 to 100 times per minute, repeating the cycle four to five times a minute.

*If you are trained in CPR, it is most likely that you would be performing mouth-to-mouth breathing on friends or loved ones and, therefore, the risk of contracting an infectious disease (such as AIDS) is minimal. However, trained rescue personnel should follow the guidelines for wearing protective resuscitation equipment that have been provided by their institution.
Source: Reproduced with permission. American Heart Association World Wide Web site http://www.amhrt.org/Heart/CPR/cpr_broch.html. Copyright American Heart Association.

◆

Q: You mentioned angina earlier. Is angina a form of heart disease?
A: No. Angina pectoris is another name for the chest pain experienced by some people with CAD. Angina is

an important warning sign that you may be at risk for a heart attack due to the buildup of plaque in your coronary arteries. The pain or discomfort of angina usually flares up when your body is under physical or emotional strain. Shoveling snow or doing yard work, getting laid off from work or arguing with your spouse, even exposure to unusually hot or cold temperatures—any of these things can trigger a bout of angina. It is under circumstances such as these that the heart must work harder to meet the increased oxygen demands of the body. When your body is straining or your emotions are running high, your heart must increase its output in order to keep pace. A healthy heart has no trouble increasing its pumping power in response to moderate or even vigorous activities (consider the strain put on the heart by a marathon runner or Olympic athlete). But when your heart's arteries are clogged and the amount of blood reaching the organ is reduced, the powerful pump on the left side of your heart cannot operate as efficiently. Your heart needs more blood at times like these, but your coronary arteries cannot comply. Specifically, angina pain is caused by an excess of lactic acid in heart tissue. Why the acidity? When the heart is starved for oxygen due to a reduced supply of incoming blood, it is unable to burn the fats it usually uses as fuel. It resorts to burning glucose (blood sugar) instead. This second-choice combustion process does not require oxygen but produces unwanted levels of lactic acid as a byproduct. Angina, which strikes over 7 million Americans, is your body's way of telling you that your heart is not getting the amount of blood that it needs due to clogged coronary arteries. The pain of angina usually fades once you are at rest or your emotions have subsided.

Q: What is variant angina?

A: Most people who suffer from angina experience the "typical" variety described above—the type that flares up during physical or mental stress. But others suffer the same sort of chest pain only while *resting*. This is variant angina pectoris, also called Prinzmetal's angina. People with coronary artery spasm often experience this type of chest pain. These are typically young men who smoke heavily. Coronary artery spasm occurs when the layer of muscle in one of the heart's arteries undergoes an involuntary contraction. (As you saw in Chapter 1, arteries do have muscles.) These contractions can impede or even halt blood flow to a portion of the heart. A severe spasm can trigger a heart attack. These spasms can occur in arteries that are clogged with plaque buildup but can also occur in healthy arteries. Over 60% of people with coronary artery spasm have severe atherosclerosis in at least one artery leading to the heart. In people with clogged arteries, the spasms usually occur near the site of plaque. Why these spasms occur at all is still something of a puzzle to doctors. While typical angina is triggered by "overdoing it," variant angina almost always flares up between midnight and 8 A.M. These attacks can be very painful and wake you from sleep. Many people with variant angina go through a brief phase of several months when the problem is most severe. It is during this "active" phase that variant angina attacks are most frequent and the risk of heart attack is greatest. About one in three people with variant angina experience heart attacks during this phase—the majority are nonfatal. After this period, most people with variant angina stabilize. The problem then tends to diminish with time and the risk of heart attack decreases.

Q: What is congestive heart failure?

A: Congestive heart failure (CHF) occurs when the heart is unable to pump enough blood to serve the needs of the body. A variety of factors can weaken the heart muscle and contribute to the development of CHF. The heart may become weakened by tissue damage suffered during a heart attack. Clogged coronary arteries or uncontrolled hypertension may fatigue the organ by increasing its workload. Congenital heart defects and diseases or infections affecting the heart muscle or its valves can also make the heart's task of pushing adequate amounts of blood through thousands of miles of blood vessels more difficult. The resulting weak blood flow causes congestion in tissues as blood returning to the heart via the veins "backs up." Working overtime in order to compensate, the heart often becomes enlarged and thickened. The kidneys, which cannot operate properly when the heart is functioning poorly, are unable to get rid of excess water and this adds to the accumulation of fluid. Congestion in the lungs can interfere with breathing, causing shortness of breath. Fluid can also accumulate in the legs, feet, and ankles, causing them to swell. As you saw in Chapter 1, blood making its way back to the heart through the veins of the legs has its work cut out for it even when the heart is working at full steam. CHF, which often results in severe fatigue, affects over 4 million Americans and is one the major reasons why people over age 65 are admitted into hospitals. About 10% of people with mild CHF and 50% of people with advanced stages of the disease die each year.

Q: What are the symptoms of CHF?

A: Symptoms include shortness of breath, swelling in the legs and feet, profound fatigue, coughing, and nausea.

Q: How is CHF treated?
A: In addition to diet and lifestyle changes, your doctor will treat any underlying medical conditions that may be causing or aggravating CHF. These include hypertension, heart rhythm irregularities, and valve defects. Medications such as digoxin (Digitalis) may be used to strengthen the heart. Other drugs such as angiotensin-converting enzyme (ACE) inhibitors or beta blockers can help reduce the heart's workload by dilating arteries. Diuretics (agents that increase urination) encourage the kidneys to expel salt and fluid, reducing the fluid buildup associated with CHF. Surgery may also be used to clear clogged coronary arteries and improve the blood flow to the heart.

Q: What does stroke have to do with cardiovascular disease?
A: We saw earlier in this chapter how an obstruction in a coronary artery can lead to a heart attack. The process leading up to a stroke is remarkably similar. Stroke occurs when an artery feeding the *brain* with oxygen and nutrients becomes obstructed by a clot or bursts and bleeds into surrounding tissue. Either way, the brain cells in the affected area are starved for oxygen within minutes. The death or damaging of these cells means that they can no longer carry out their functions. The consequences of a stroke depend on which cells are affected and to what extent. A stroke can result in speech problems, paralysis, and loss of memory or reasoning ability. The effects of a stroke are usually permanent because dead brain cells cannot be replaced or repaired. Sometimes other parts of the brain are able to "take over" for the affected cells, and the victims of stroke can recover some of the skills or abilities lost immediately after the

attack. In the most serious cases, stroke results in coma or death. Almost 600,000 Americans each year suffer these "brain attacks." About 150,000 die as a result of stroke and many more live with some form of disability. Most strokes (70% to 80%) occur when an artery leading to the brain is blocked by a thrombus. These clots usually form at the site of atherosclerotic plaque buildup. This type of stroke usually occurs when blood pressure is at its lowest—late at night or early in the morning—because it is easier for a clot to plug an artery when the stream of blood offers least resistance. Strokes due to a thrombus are often preceded by a transient ischemic attack (TIA). The symptoms of a TIA, also called a ministroke, are similar to those of a full-blown brain attack except that they only last from a few minutes to a half hour. You can think of a TIA as your brain's version of angina—a warning sign that you are at risk for a stroke.

Q: How would I know if I were having a stroke or TIA? What are the symptoms?
A: You should seek help immediately if you experience any of these symptoms, which may indicate a stroke or TIA. Keep in mind that you will not see all of these symptoms in every incidence of stroke. In the case of TIA, these signs will be temporary.

- Weakness in an arm, hand, or leg
- Numbness in one side of the face or body
- Inability to see out of one eye
- Difficulty speaking
- Difficulty comprehending what someone is saying
- Sudden onset of a severe headache
- Dizziness or loss of balance

Q: Can a stroke occur for other reasons?
A: Yes. Some strokes are caused by an embolus that lodges in an artery leading to the brain. An embolus is a blood clot that is "on the move." Originating in a coronary or other artery, an embolus may travel through the bloodstream until it reaches one of the arteries feeding the brain, where it becomes firmly lodged. A smaller number of strokes are caused by ruptured blood vessels in the brain. This type of stroke is far less common than the others but is more deadly. When a blood vessel bursts in the brain, it may bleed into the space between the brain and skull or into the brain tissue itself—in both of these scenarios, the brain cells that rely on the ruptured vessel for blood are deprived. Major causes of stroke include uncontrolled hypertension, smoking, and heart disease.

◆

Putting Your Heart to the Test

In addition to checking blood pressure, developing a cholesterol profile, and sometimes taking plain old X rays, your doctor may recommend any of a growing number of tests and imaging procedures designed to evaluate your cardiovascular health. The general rule of thumb? Doctors usually start with the most basic procedures and then employ those that are more invasive (penetrating) if necessary. Some common or important tests used to detect and evaluate CAD, heart rhythm irregularities, or structural problems affecting the heart are listed on the following pages.

Noninvasive (Nonpenetrating) Tests

Electrocardiogram (ECG or EKG)

The graph line produced by an ECG is familiar to most people through movies or TV hospital dramas—the term *flat-lining* has even entered America's vocabulary as a metaphor for life's end. In the real world, an ECG is an important tool used by doctors to record the electrical activity of the heart and produce a visual representation of what a heartbeat looks like. An ECG, which involves placing electrode patches on the arms, legs, and chest, is used to assess heart muscle damage or enlargement as well as abnormal hearth rhythms such as arrhythmias. A signal average electrocardiogram (SAE), which uses computers to enhance the signal, is basically like an ECG except that it records more information and takes longer to conduct.

Exercise Stress Test

This test is used to evaluate heart function while you exercise by walking or jogging on a treadmill or pedaling a stationary bike. Your heartbeat is recorded on an ECG to see how your heart responds to physical exertion. A stress test can help to determine if your heart is getting insufficient blood (due to clogged arteries, for example) and can evaluate what level of exercise is safe for someone with heart disease. Breathing rate and blood-pressure level may also be monitored as part of the test. As you will see below, a stress test is sometimes combined with an imaging procedure in order to provide more information about how well the heart is functioning.

Echocardiogram

This procedure, which does not involve radiation, uses sound waves to create an image of the inside of the heart. An echocardiogram can reveal the shape and motion of the heart's four chambers and valves. It is usually performed while you are at rest but can also be used to evaluate your heart after you have exercised on a treadmill or stationary bike.

Holter Monitor

Think of this as your own portable ECG. You can wear this small, battery-powered unit for a day or two while it records the electrical activity of your heart. Your doctor evaluates the results by studying the Holter monitor's recorded tape. Ambulatory electrocardiography is another (and much longer) name for Holter monitoring.

Tilt Table Test

As its name implies, this test involves a table and some tilting. By gently securing you to a tilt table and then moving it through various angles, your doctor can determine if you are vulnerable to sudden changes in blood-pressure or pulse rate. You are connected to an ECG and blood-pressure monitor during the test.

Ultrafast CT Scan

In an ultrafast computed tomography (CT) test, you lie on a table as an X ray machine scans your chest, taking cross-sectional images of the blood vessels in your heart. The density of calcium (a component of plaque, see page 23) in the coronary arteries is an indicator of the presence of coronary atherosclerosis. The test is rapid, and some doctors believe it is a good screening to predict the occurrence of heart attack and other cardiac events.

Invasive Tests

Thallium Stress Test

This test evaluates the flow of blood to the heart by combining a stress test with a dye-enhanced imaging procedure. A small, safe amount of radioactive thallium is administered via an IV in your hand after you reach your maximum heart rate during exercise on a treadmill or stationary bike. X rays of the heart and blood vessels are then taken by a special camera that encircles you as you lie flat on an imaging table. The thallium-laced blood reaching the heart via the coronary arteries shows up on these X rays and reveals how much blood is reaching the heart. If your arteries are healthy and free of plaque buildup, all areas of the heart will be highlighted by the thallium. If these arteries are narrowed by atherosclerosis, certain areas of the heart may appear to be "missing" on the X rays—in other words, they do not appear on the images due to the fact that clogged arteries prevented the dye from reaching its destination in the heart. Additional X rays are taken several hours later in order to evaluate blood flow to the heart while you are at rest. Note: Large breasts in women can sometimes absorb too much of the tracer and prevent proper amounts from reaching the heart even when the coronary arteries are clear.

Catheter Procedures

Procedures involving catheters (flexible, hollow tubes) can be used to identity the presence and severity of narrowed arteries and help determine the best way to treat them. These procedures, which are sometimes referred to as the "gold standard" of cardiac testing, are usually done on an outpatient basis. They require overnight fasting and mild sedation.

- In coronary angiography, a thin catheter is inserted into an artery in an arm or leg and guided into the coronary arteries. A radioactive dye is then injected into the catheter and moving X-ray images are taken. These images, which you and your doctor can view on an overhead TV monitor, map the route taken by the dye through the coronary arteries and the heart.

- Cerebral angiography is similar to the procedure described immediately above except that it is used to detect atherosclerosis in the main arteries supplying the brain, not the heart, with blood.

Note: In the elderly and people with advanced heart disease, there is a very slight risk that a catheter procedure will trigger a heart attack or stroke.

Transesophageal Echocardiogram (TEE)

This version of an echocardiogram provides clearer images of the heart than its noninvasive (nonpenetrating) namesake. In a TEE (a minimally invasive procedure), the transducer, which emits and receives the sounds waves, is placed nearer to the heart by inserting it into the esophagus (the tube connecting the mouth to the stomach) via the throat.

◆

Knowing Your Risk Factors and Preventing Heart Disease

Susan, age 58, is a retiree who teaches writing part time. She also volunteers teaching crafts to seniors at the local nursing home and is heavily involved in the lives of her two grandchildren. As a busy post-menopausal woman only slightly over her ideal weight, Susan was a little surprised when I told her the results of her lipid (fat) profile. Her total cholesterol and low-density lipoprotein (LDL) cholesterol levels were slightly elevated. Her level of high-density lipoprotein (HDL) was on the low side and her triglycerides were elevated. Susan was surprised to learn that in the five or ten years after menopause women suffer from heart disease almost as often as men of the same age and are actually more likely to have elevated blood cholesterol. Most doctors speculate that lower estrogen levels after menopause are what make women more vulnerable to cardiovascular disease as they get older. I told Susan that together we could reduce her risk of heart disease by lowering her LDL cholesterol and triglyceride levels and raising her HDL levels. Why worry about triglycerides? Studies suggest that elevated levels of this blood fat are an important risk factor for atherosclerosis (narrowing and hardening of the arteries) in postmenopausal women.

Susan and I reviewed the types of foods she was eating and how much exercise she was getting and decided that she needed to increase her level of aerobic activities and decrease her intake of saturated fats. Susan began walking to and from her writing class instead of taking the bus, and she started taking a swimming class twice a week at the local community center. She also made adjustments in the amount of saturated fat she was eating. These diet and lifestyle modifications improved Susan's lipid profile, and we decided to watch in the future to see if she was a good candidate for hormone replacement therapy (HRT) to reduce her cardiovascular risk through estrogen supplementation and to build bone if Susan was at risk for osteoporosis. For now, however, Susan is opting not to go on HRT because of the slightly increased risk for breast cancer that HRT poses and because a bone scan revealed that she is not at risk for osteoporosis.

What types of exercise help to protect against heart disease and how often should I work out? What can I do to keep my blood pressure under control? Can aspirin really be used to prevent a heart attack? As a cardiologist, these are the sorts of questions that I enjoy answering. They give me an opportunity to explain practical ways that people can keep their cardiovascular systems healthy and have fewer heart attacks and strokes. The really good news about heart disease is that most of us can prevent it and in some cases even reverse it. While there are no quick fixes, this chapter and the next focus on lifestyle changes that you can start making today in order to keep your heart healthy for a lifetime. These include eliminating smoking and other unhealthy habits, eating a proper diet and getting regular exercise, maintaining an ideal weight, and managing medical conditions such as hypertension (high blood pressure) and diabetes. Heeding some of the advice offered in these two chapters may also improve your general health and sense of well-being. Trimming the fat from your diet, for example, not only helps to prevent heart attack and stroke but can also improve self-image. Tired of being winded after climbing a flight of stairs or running a short distance to hail a cab? Exercise helps to condition your heart and lungs and may lift your mood and melt away stress. Adopting a heart-healthy lifestyle also sets a great example for the youngest members of your family. We must remember that our children see in us examples of how to live—whether we like it or not. One of the most important health lessons we can teach our children is how to keep their hearts healthy and strong.

Q: I want to take charge of my health. What are some of the risk factors for heart disease that I can change?

A: A variety of factors can affect your risk. Some of these you can change and some you cannot. If you have risk factors for heart disease that cannot be changed, it is especially important to take steps to minimize those that are under your control. See Risk Factors for Heart Disease That You Cannot Change on page 51 for other factors that contribute to the development of heart and blood vessel disease.

- *Cholesterol levels.* Is it better to have a high cholesterol level or a low one? That depends on *which* kind of cholesterol is being measured. Doctors measure blood cholesterol in several ways to determine who is at risk for heart disease and heart attack. A high level of total cholesterol or low-density lipoprotein (LDL) cholesterol (the so-called "bad" cholesterol) puts you at increased risk. When it comes to HDL cholesterol, higher is usually better. See Chapter 4 for more information about cholesterol levels and fat.

- *Smoking.* Cigarette smoke can harden arteries and thicken the blood in the 50 million Americans who smoke. Smokers are twice as likely to suffer heart attacks as nonsmokers and are more likely to die from an attack. Nonsmokers exposed to secondhand cigarette smoke may also be at increased risk for heart disease. Smoking pipes or cigars also appears to increase the risk of cardiovascular disease.

- *Hypertension.* If not properly controlled, hypertension (high blood pressure) damages the inner linings of arteries and sets the stage for atherosclerosis and the development of CAD. Hypertension also increases the risk of stroke.

- *Exercise.* Getting 30 minutes of aerobic exercise on most days of the week can help prevent heart disease and improve your overall health. Hundreds of thousands of Americans die each year as a result of a sedentary lifestyle.

- *Weight.* Obesity (an excess of body fat that equals 20% or more of your ideal weight) can contribute to the development of CAD, heart attack, and stroke. Carrying around extra pounds puts unnecessary strain on the heart and makes the organ work harder than it would have to if your body were leaner. Obesity raises total cholesterol and triglyceride levels and reduces the amount of HDL cholesterol in the blood. Being overweight also contributes to the development of several other risk factors for heart disease, including hypertension and diabetes. See Chapter 5 for more information on obesity.

- *Estrogen.* As the primary female sex hormone, estrogen helps to keep the cardiovascular system healthy and prevent heart disease in women. After the age of 50, which is typically considered postmenopause and is also when estrogen levels drop, heart disease rates in women climb. Many doctors believe that these increased heart disease rates are related to the loss of estrogen.
- *Triglycerides.* Most of the fat in your body is stored in a form known as triglycerides. See Chapter 5 for information on how high triglyceride levels (200 mg/dL or over) may contribute to the development of CAD.
- *Stress.* Some studies suggest a link between the risk of CAD and high levels of emotional stress. Doctors are not certain exactly how stress increases the risk of heart disease. Does it do so directly by way of some as yet unknown mechanism or does stress only affect the development of other risk factors? People who are regularly under stress, for example, may be more likely to overeat or smoke to relieve tension and are more likely to have hypertension. If you feel that you are often stressed out, ask your doctor about relaxation techniques such as meditation or yoga.

Q: I've been trying to get my husband to stop smoking for several years. Can you explain why quitting is so important?

A: I would be happy to, especially since there are so many great reasons why he and 50 million other American smokers should kick the habit. Most doctors agree that smoking is the *single most preventable* cause of death in the United States. As most of us probably know by now, smoking is associated with heart disease, lung and other cancers, and a variety of other health problems. It is certainly one of the most important risk factors for cardiovascular disease, contributing to about 350,000 heart disease deaths each year in this country alone. Smoking leads directly to the buildup of plaque deposits in arteries, dramatically increases the risk of heart attack, and plays a central role in the development of other heart disease risk factors such as hypertension. Consider this sobering statistic: People who smoke are *twice* as likely to suffer heart attacks as are nonsmokers! Even light smokers are significantly at risk for life-threatening disease. In one recent study of 13,000 men conducted over a period of 25 years, those who smoked fewer than ten cigarettes a day (less than half a pack) had a 30% higher risk of death due to heart disease or lung cancer than nonsmokers. Cigar smokers are equally at risk for these diseases; in fact, the National Cancer Institute reported recently that although cigar smokers inhale less smoke than cigarette smokers, cigars are equal in toxicity to cigarettes because they contain up to 90 times as much of some carcinogens as cigarettes. Not only are smokers more likely to die from heart attacks but they are likely to die faster (within one hour), cheating themselves out of crucial minutes or hours that may save their lives. As you saw in Chapter 2, the key to surviving a heart attack depends on recognizing the symptoms early and receiving swift medical attention. Because smokers have a smaller window of survival time once a heart attack begins, they may not live long enough for an emergency medical services (EMS) team to arrive on the scene and administer lifesaving care.

The fact that your husband smokes may have some serious health consequences for you as well. Even non-smokers routinely exposed to cigarette or cigar smoke are more likely to die from cardiovascular disease. Studies suggest that regular exposure to secondhand smoke may double the risk of heart disease and cause up to 40,000 heart attack deaths a year in the United States. What other bad health habit can you think of that has the power to kill its onlookers? This sort of exposure may occur if you live with a smoker or frequent bars or other nightspots that permit smoking. To protect your health and that of other nonsmokers in your family, make your home a nonsmoking zone and ask your husband to smoke elsewhere until he kicks the habit. This will help to protect your children from being exposed to deadly cigarette smoke and to the unhealthy example being set by your husband.

◆

A Question for Smokers

Most smokers are unaware of the damage wreaked by cigarette smoke on their hearts and blood vessels (flexible tubes that carry blood through the body). Once you have read this chapter and learn how destructive cigarettes are to your heart's health, you owe it to yourself to answer the question, "Is smoking really worth it?" Millions of American men and women over the last few decades have responded with *no*. More than 40% of Americans were smoking in 1965—a little less than half the population of the United States! Today that number has dropped to 25%. While nicotine addiction is one of the most difficult to break, there have never been so many different ways to quit smoking or good reasons to do it. Your doctor has a variety of smoking cessation techniques that can help you kick the habit for good. Now is the time! Join the swelling ranks of the 1.3 million smokers in America who quit each year.

◆

Q: Exactly how does smoking cause CAD and heart attack?

A: Each cigarette that a person smokes launches an all-out attack on the heart and blood vessels, causing damage in a variety of ways. The nicotine and carbon monoxide in cigarette smoke both encourage the buildup of plaque in the arteries. Smoking also reduces the amount of oxygen reaching the heart and other parts of your body and thickens the blood so that it is more likely to form an artery-blocking clot. Carbon monoxide, the same noxious gas found in car exhaust, damages the smooth inner surface of coronary and other arteries. This damage encourages the buildup of plaque on artery walls and makes them hard and narrow, allowing less oxygen-laden blood to reach the heart or brain. But carbon monoxide deprives your body of oxygen in other ways as well—namely by attaching itself to red blood cells. As you saw in Chapter 1, red blood cells are the cellular vehicles that carry oxygen from the lungs and deliver it to the heart and other tissue throughout the body. The carbon monoxide that enters your bloodstream while smoking is unwelcome cargo. These gas molecules hitch a ride on red blood cells, occupying valuable space that is normally reserved for the oxygen on which your body depends. In addition to narrowing arteries and taking the place of oxygen in your blood, cigarette smoke thickens the blood itself by boosting levels of fibrinogen (a substance that tends to make blood clot). Thicker blood, in turn, increases the likelihood that a blood clot (called a thrombus) will form near the site of a plaque eruption— the result is often a heart attack or stroke. If all this were not enough, smoking has also been shown to reduce levels of high-density lipoprotein (HDL) cholesterol—the so-called "good" cholesterol that lowers your risk of heart disease when present in sufficient amounts.

Q: What does blood pressure have to do with heart disease?

A: The pressure of your blood is one of the factors that determine the health of your heart and vessels. As you saw in Chapter 1, blood pressure is the force that your blood exerts on the walls of blood vessels, arteries, and veins. All the blood in your body is under pressure to one degree or another but this pressure is not the same everywhere. The blood pressure that doctors measure is that present in your arteries, the large vessels that carry blood away from the heart. While the system composed of your heart and blood vessels is designed to work best within a certain range of pressure, it can accommodate inevitable fluctuations that result from emotional stress or physical exertion. Watching your favorite vase tumble off the mantel and shatter on the floor or sitting for hours in rush-hour traffic can temporarily boost pressure, as can feats of strength or speed on the athletic field. It is when blood pressure stays high all the time that it begins to damage arteries leading to the heart and brain. When healthy, these arteries have a smooth inner surface that encourages the flow of blood. The prolonged strain imposed on the circulatory system by consistently high blood pressure can actually damage the inner linings of arteries and make them rougher. Plaque deposits are more likely to develop in the areas of damage that result from uncontrolled hypertension. If untreated, hypertension also can increase the heart's workload to the point that the organ becomes enlarged and weakened over time. High blood pressure is a major risk factor for CAD and heart attack as well as stroke, especially when combined with other risk factors.

◆

Risk Factors for Heart Disease That You Cannot Change

Earlier in the chapter we discussed the risk factors that you can change. Other factors, from age and race to diabetes, may also contribute to the development of cardiovascular disease.

- *Age.* While atherosclerosis (hardening of the arteries) usually starts to develop in childhood or young adulthood, most people who die as a result of CAD are age 65 or older (slightly more of them are men than women).
- *Gender.* Men suffer heart attacks earlier in life than women and are more likely to die from heart disease at any age. Older women who have heart attacks are twice as likely to die from them within a few weeks than are men of the same age.
- *Race.* Blacks have a greater risk of cardiovascular disease than whites. Though blacks are less at risk for CAD, they are more likely to suffer strokes due to the fact that blacks as a group are two to three times more likely to have hypertension. Blacks tend to develop high blood pressure earlier in life and usually experience a more severe form.

- **Heredity.** Heart disease tends to run in families and is influenced by genetic factors. Your risk of heart disease is higher if you have a first-degree relative (mother, father, or sibling) who developed the disease before age 55. People genetically predisposed to high cholesterol levels are most at risk. But genes are probably not the whole story. Doctors also suspect that some children in families affected by heart disease increase their risk by adopting the bad health habits (also known as transmissible risks) of their parents. Parents who do not exercise, for example, or who regularly serve high-fat foods at the dinner table may be sending the wrong message to their kids about the importance of heart health.

- **Diabetes.** Over 80% of people with diabetes die as a result of cardiovascular disease. People with diabetes are either unable to produce adequate amounts of insulin or cannot use the hormone properly to convert glucose (blood sugar) into energy. The metabolic process that is part of diabetes is associated with increased triglyceride levels and lower HDL levels, which are risk factors for atherosclerosis, CAD, heart attack, and stroke.

◆

Q: What causes high blood pressure and how can it be controlled?

A: Over 50 million Americans live with some degree of hypertension, though many are unaware that they are affected by high blood pressure because it rarely causes symptoms that you can see or feel. That is why it is so important to have your blood pressure checked by your doctor at least once every two years even if you believe that your pressure is within normal limits. Hypertension sometimes occurs as a result of congenital (present at birth) heart defects or kidney or other health problems. In essential hypertension, which accounts for over 90% of cases, the cause is unknown. A number of factors can contribute to the development of hypertension or worsen the condition. High blood pressure tends to run in families and is more likely to strike those who are middle-aged or older. Blacks are several times more likely to suffer from hypertension than are whites, and blacks tend to develop elevated blood pressure at a younger age. Hypertension also occurs more frequently in the following groups: people who do not exercise, obese people, heavy drinkers, women who take oral contraceptives, and people with underlying medical conditions such as diabetes, kidney disease, or gout. Many people with hypertension can control their blood-pressure levels by maintaining an ideal weight, restricting the amount of sodium they consume (2,400 mg a day is the upper limit), and getting more exercise. Studies also show that a diet that is rich in fruits, vegetables, and low-fat dairy foods and that is also low in saturated fat, total fat, and cholesterol can lower blood pressure even if an ideal body weight is not maintained and sodium intake is not reduced. A diet that is rich in fruits and vegetables alone can also lower blood pressure, although to a lesser extent. If lifestyle changes do not lower your pressure to acceptable levels after several months or if your blood pressure is very high at the time of diagnosis, your doctor may recommend prescription medication. Diuretics (agents that increase urination) are used to help rid the body of excess sodium and fluid while other drugs are sometimes taken to relax blood vessels and keep them from constricting.

See Chapter 1 for more information on blood pressure ranges.

◆

Is America Exercising Enough?

The good news is that Americans are more physically active today than they were a few decades ago. Unfortunately, most of us are still not getting as much exercise as we should, whether in our youth or our golden years.

- It is estimated that over 50% of white American men and women do not get enough aerobic exercise to protect the cardiovascular system from disease. Blacks and Hispanics exercise even less.
- Older Americans tend to work out less often than they did during their youth despite the fact that exercise, which strengthens bones and sharpens the sense of balance and coordination, is more important than ever as we age.
- Up to half of all children do not exercise on a regular basis.

◆

Q: Just how important is exercise in preventing heart disease?
A: It is hard to overestimate the role played by regular aerobic exercise. When we use the term *aerobic* we are referring to physical activities that increase heart and breathing rates and make the heart work harder to meet the increased oxygen demands of the body. From jogging and bicycling to in-line skating and skipping rope, regular aerobic workouts are a crucial component of a heart-healthy lifestyle. They not only help to condition the heart and lungs but

may also aid in managing medical conditions such as hypertension and diabetes, and they improve HDL blood cholesterol levels. A program of regular exercise, which should include a balance of aerobic and weight-bearing activities (such as weight-lifting), can also help to prevent numerous health problems affecting our bodies and minds. (Weight-bearing exercise is important for strengthening bones and building muscle.) Physical activity should be a routine part of our lives from childhood to our most advanced years. It is estimated that 10% of all deaths in the United States are the result of a sedentary lifestyle.

To protect the cardiovascular system from disease, most doctors recommend that you get about 30 minutes of aerobic exercise on most days of the week. At least three days a week of heart-pumping exercise is necessary to provide significant cardiovascular benefit. The key is to find activities that you can do on a regular basis. Even the best exercises are of little use if you lack the time or inclination to do them. With a little experimenting you will discover exercises that are right for you. The fact is there have never been so many fun ways to stay in shape. Exercise is a lot more than just lifting barbells or jogging endless miles on a treadmill—though both these activities are excellent ways to build muscle and stay in shape. Skating, mountain biking, swimming, cross-country skiing, brisk walking, jumping rope, aerobic dancing, and hiking are just some of the exercises that help to condition the heart and lungs. Exercises like these are a great way to prevent atherosclerosis, trim the fat from your waistline, boost blood levels of good cholesterol, lower triglycerides, and manage hypertension and diabetes—the list of benefits goes on and on. But before you head off to the running track or an aerobics class, talk to your doctor about the exercise program you plan to start. Your doctor can explain how to get the most out of your workout and how to exercise safely. If you have risk factors for CAD, your doctor may wish to give you an exercise stress test to evaluate the health of your heart and determine what level of exertion is safe for you. Chapter 2 for information on exercise stress tests and other ways that doctors diagnose heart and blood vessel diseases.

◆
Getting More Exercise Out of Your Daily Life

Even when you are not officially "working out," a few simple tips can help you stay more physically active around the house or even during work hours. The tips provided below are designed to get you started. Once you get into the habit of being more physically active, you will think of additional ways to stay fit outside of the gym.

At Home

- Housework and yard work are great ways to improve the look of your home and get some exercise in the process.
- Take a brisk walk before breakfast or after dinner (or both). Work your way up to 30 minutes per walk.
- Walk or bike to the corner store instead of driving.
- Spend a few minutes pedaling on your stationary bicycle while watching TV.
- Volunteer to walk the dog instead of finding excuses to avoid it.
- Do not always take the parking spot nearest the entrance to your local shopping mall or department store—walk the extra distance. Take a few extra "window shopping" laps around the mall.

At Work

- Take a walk with a coworker while brainstorming new ideas or working out problems.
- Walk down the hall to speak to another employee instead of reaching for the telephone or intercom.
- Skip the elevator and take the stairs. If your workplace is located on one of the higher floors, take the elevator part of the way and then use the stairs.
- Stay at hotels with fitness centers or swimming pools while on business trips.
- Take along a jump rope in your suitcase when you travel and use it in your hotel room. (Keep in mind that jumping rope is a strenuous activity and you should be in good physical condition if you plan to do it.)
- Participate in or start a recreation league at your company. Form a sports team to raise money for charity events.
- Walk around your building during a break or your lunch hour.
- Get off the bus a few blocks early and walk the rest of the way to work or home.

Source: American Heart Association.

◆

Q: What is diabetes and how does it contribute to heart disease?
A: People with diabetes mellitus either have difficulty producing insulin or develop a resistance to the hormone, depending on which form of the disease they have. Insulin causes glucose to enter cells, which results in the

intracellular processes that include the production of energy. Insulin also regulates the way your body absorbs and stores other nutrients and fat that you get from food. Type 1 diabetes, which is also called juvenile-onset diabetes or insulin-dependent diabetes, is the less common of the two types and is usually diagnosed before age 20. In this often inherited form of the disease, the pancreas is not able to produce sufficient amounts of insulin. Most Americans with diabetes have type 2, which is also called adult-onset diabetes or noninsulin-dependent diabetes. While 16 million Americans are believed to have type 2 diabetes, only about half that number have been diagnosed with the disease. In this form of diabetes, which usually occurs after age 40, the body is able to make insulin but has trouble using it properly. Both forms of diabetes significantly increase the risk of developing CAD, heart attack, and stroke because the disease can cause damage in arteries that supply the heart or brain with blood (as well as blood vessels in the eyes and other parts of the body). The metabolic process that is part of diabetes is associated with increased triglyceride levels and lower HDL levels, which are risk factors for atherosclerosis, CAD, heart attack, and stroke. People with type 2 diabetes tend to be overweight or obese as well. Just how much impact does diabetes have on heart disease risk? About 80% of people with diabetes die of some form of cardiovascular disease. This statistic emphasizes the importance of diagnosing the disease and beginning treatment before the damage caused by diabetes becomes extensive.

The symptoms of both forms of diabetes are similar. They include severe thirst, unexplained weight loss, frequent urination, blurred vision, fatigue, and frequent infections of the urinary tract or vagina. In addition to these symptoms, people with type 2 diabetes may have extra fat in the abdominal area or experience episodes of erectile dysfunction (more commonly known as impotence). While there is no cure for diabetes, a strict dietary regimen—which includes avoiding simple sugars such as cane sugar and those found in honey and fruit juices—combined with an exercise program can be effective at controlling glucose levels. People with type 1 diabetes also rely on long-term insulin therapy to manage their condition. The treatment of type 2 diabetes often consists of lifestyle changes alone but occasionally requires the use of blood sugar–lowering drugs such as sulfonylureas, metformin (Glucophage), acarbose (Precose), and thiazolidinediones (for example, troglitazone [Rezulin]). It is especially important for people with diabetes to avoid smoking and control hypertension. In addition to heart disease, diabetes is associated with kidney disorders, blindness, and nerve damage.

Q: What does estrogen have to do with CAD?

A: The loss of estrogen during menopause occurs coincidentally with an increased risk of CAD, and many doctors believe it is a cause of heart disease. This hormone is produced mainly in the ovaries and plays an important role in maintaining the health of the cardiovascular system in women. By connecting to communication ports (called receptors) located on the surfaces of cells, estrogen delivers chemical "messages" that affect blood fat levels and the inner surfaces of arteries, where plaque tends to develop. Estrogen appears to boost HDL levels, prevent the buildup of plaque on artery walls, and wash away fatty deposits by increasing blood flow. Some women take supplemental estrogen after menopause to help fight heart disease, avoid bone-weakening osteoporosis, and help control troublesome menopausal symptoms such as hot flashes and vaginal dryness. Estrogen replacement therapy (ERT) consists of estrogen alone while hormone replacement therapy (HRT) is a combination of estrogen and progestin (a synthetic version of another important female hormone called progesterone). Women who take supplemental estrogen after menopause may reduce their risk of heart disease by as much as 50%. Selective estrogen receptor modulator (SERM) medications such as raloxifene (Evista) may also help to prevent heart disease in postmenopausal women by mimicking the effects of estrogen. See Chapter 8 for more information on the connection between estrogen and heart disease.

Q: Can aspirin really help to prevent heart attacks?

A: Yes. Aspirin is not just for headaches anymore. Thanks to its ability to prevent blood clots and stabilize plaque deposits, this nonsteroidal anti-inflammatory drug (NSAID) is now being used by some Americans with CAD to prevent the risk of heart attack and stroke. If you have already suffered a heart attack, aspirin may reduce your risk of having another by over 30%. This analgesic (pain reliever) can also reduce the risk of a stroke in someone who has had one before or experienced only a transient ischemic attack (TIA)—a "ministroke" that often precedes a full-blown brain attack. How does aspirin work its wonders? As you saw in Chapter 2, a heart attack or stroke is usually triggered by the rupturing of a plaque deposit in an artery leading to the heart or brain. This is often followed by the formation of a blood clot at or near the site of the rupture that effectively seals off the artery and prevents blood from reaching its destination and delivering its oxygen cargo. Aspirin helps to prevent these blood clots from forming by affecting special cells in the blood called platelets. These sticky, irregularly shaped cells routinely rush to the scene of an injury or wound and clump together to help seal off the injured area and stop the bleeding. Most of the time we are grateful for the action of platelets. They save our lives on a regular basis by preventing us from bleeding to death. But when platelets arrive on the scene of a ruptured plaque deposit within an artery, they can become killers. Aspirin works as a clot buster by stopping these platelets from sticking together and forming a seal that blocks the flow of blood. Aspirin's anti-inflammatory properties may also help to preempt heart attacks and strokes. Studies have shown that plaque deposits sometimes rupture after the area containing the plaque becomes inflamed. This inflammation can actually weaken the plaque, rendering it unstable and more likely to break apart. By reducing inflammation, aspirin may have a stabilizing effect on plaque and help to prevent ruptures.

Studies in men have shown that taking 325 mg of coated aspirin every day is a good form of secondary prevention for those who already have heart disease. For those who want to practice primary prevention, 325 mg of coated aspirin every other day is an acceptable dosage. If you do not have heart disease and are considering taking aspirin as a form of primary prevention, go over your risk factors with your doctor. Too much aspirin can thin the blood drastically and lead to unwanted side effects such as gastrointestinal (GI) irritation or the formation of stomach ulcers. If you are considering starting on aspirin therapy, talk to your doctor first. Your doctor can help you decide which dosage (if any) is right for you and how long you should continue to take aspirin. Aspirin may not be recommended if you have kidney or liver disease, peptic ulcer disease or other GI problems, or bleeding disorders. Be sure to inform your doctor if you drink heavily or are already taking other blood-thinning medications. Aspirin can also increase the risk of bleeding after an operation or dental surgery, so always inform your doctor that you are on aspirin therapy before scheduling any such procedure.

Understanding Cholesterol

Todd is a 25-year-old word processor and struggling
actor who is always on the go. Although he has time to
work out at a gym three times a week, he rarely has time to
cook or eat well-balanced meals and often finds that he
is eating at fast-food restaurants. On a routine checkup
that included a cholesterol screening, he discovered that
his total cholesterol level was 280, his low-density lipoprotein (LDL) cholesterol level—also called "bad"
cholesterol—was high and his high-density lipoprotein
(HDL) cholesterol level—also called "good" cholesterol—
was quite low.

Todd felt in great shape, but in examining his family
history I discovered that heart disease and high cholesterol levels ran in his family. I reviewed his diet with him,
and we came up with a plan to lower his intake of saturated fats by increasing his intake of fruits and vegetables

and substituting leaner cuts of meats and low-fat dairy food for the cheeseburgers and french fries that were a large part of his diet. Since Todd was already exercising regularly, he merely needed to keep up his current exercise routine while he adjusted his diet.

I also explained to Todd how high cholesterol levels and high LDL and low HDL levels can lead to atherosclerosis and heart disease. We also discussed the hereditary aspects of this disease—his grandfather had died of a heart attack at the age of 55 and his father had high cholesterol levels. I explained that this placed Todd at a greater risk for high cholesterol than other people had, and that by adjusting his diet and monitoring his cholesterol levels he could most probably avoid serious heart disease.

After several months on his new diet, Todd was quite pleased to find that his total cholesterol level had decreased and his LDL/HDL ratio had improved significantly. At his checkup, Todd remarked that the changes in his diet had not been that hard to do and that he enjoyed many of the new foods he was eating. He was told to keep up his routine and that his cholesterol levels would be monitored periodically.

Cholesterol has had a high profile in the health-conscious previous decade. From cereals to bran muffins, grocery store shelves are stocked with foods advertising themselves as cholesterol-free or claiming to lower your cholesterol levels. These days, coworkers standing around the water cooler are almost as likely to be discussing their cholesterol levels as last night's sports scores or rumors of office romance. This increased awareness of cholesterol and its role in heart health comes as good news to doctors. As you saw in Chapter 2, cholesterol is a major building block of the plaque that can accumulate in your arteries and ultimately lead to a heart attack or stroke. That is why measurements of cholesterol in the blood are such important factors in determining who is at risk for heart disease. Your cholesterol level is not just affected by the amount of cholesterol contained in the foods you eat. It is also influenced for better or worse by the amount of saturated and unsaturated fat in your diet. These dietary fats are known as triglycerides and are discussed in Chapter 5. An understanding of cholesterol and dietary fats and their role in cardiovascular health is important for men and women of all ages. While America's collective cholesterol count has undergone a healthy reduction in recent decades, many of us still need to lower our levels of this blood fat (also called a blood lipid, which is composed of cholesterol and triglyceride) in order to prevent coronary artery disease (CAD). It is estimated that a little over half of all Americans have elevated cholesterol levels and one in five have high cholesterol. Though heart disease is still considered a man's problem by some, women tend to suffer from high cholesterol more often than men after age 55. More than 35% of American teens have borderline-high cholesterol levels that put them at risk for heart disease later in life. This chapter discusses the factors that influence cholesterol levels and provides some general rules of thumb to help you make heart-healthy dietary choices.

Q: What is cholesterol?

A: Cholesterol is a waxy substance that is classified as a steroid. Most of us consume cholesterol on a daily basis in the foods we eat. You may be surprised to learn that even in the absence of dietary cholesterol your body manufactures a certain amount on its own. The 1,000 mg a day of cholesterol produced by the liver is really all your body needs. *Needs* is the operative word here because cholesterol plays an important role in maintaining good health. Your body uses it to make cell membranes and sex hormones. Cholesterol is also an important component of bile, which helps your body to digest food. The problem with cholesterol is that most of us have too much of it in our blood. This occurs mainly because we get too much of it through our diets and consume saturated fats that help to elevate our cholesterol levels even further. The excess cholesterol in your blood can lead to the formation of plaque in your arteries. Reducing levels of this blood fat can reduce your risk of heart disease and help prevent heart attacks and strokes.

What types of food contain cholesterol? Unfortunately, some important staples of the American diet. Cholesterol is found only in foods that come from animals—meats, poultry, fish and other seafood, and dairy products. Fruits, vegetables, grains, and nuts, and other plant foods are cholesterol-free. Foods particularly high in cholesterol include egg yolks (a single egg yolk contains over 200 mg of cholesterol), organ meats, and shrimp. You do not necessarily need to give up some of your favorite foods in order to limit your intake of cholesterol, but trimming the fat and eating them in moderation is necessary. Lean cuts of beef or pork, for example, contain about the same amount of cholesterol as lower-cholesterol sources such as chicken or fish. How much dietary cholesterol is too much? The American Heart Association (AHA) recommends that you limit your average daily intake of dietary cholesterol to 300 mg a day—and if you already have coronary artery disease (CAD) you should consume no more than 200 mg. As it stands now, American men consume about 360 mg of cholesterol daily while women get about 240 mg. Eating a diet rich in fruits and vegetables, avoiding meat or eating lean cuts of it, and reading labels to avoid high-cholesterol foods are some of the first steps you can make to reduce your dietary cholesterol and lower your risk of heart disease.

◆

A Look at the Cholesterol in Some Common Foods

Food	Cholesterol (mg)
Processed lunch meat, lean roast beef (2 oz)	17
Meatloaf (3 oz, cooked)	64
Ground beef, extra lean broiled medium (3 oz)	71
Link sausage, smoked beef and or pork (4 in. link, 1⅛ in. round)	39
Bologna (2 slices)	31
Frankfurter, cured (5 in. frank, ⅞ in. around)	33
Liverwurst (3¼ slices, ¼ in. thick, 2½ in. diameter)	87
Processed lunch meat, chicken breast (2 oz)	30
Chicken drumstick, without skin (2 drumsticks)	79
Turkey leg, with skin (3 oz)	60
Shrimp, cooked with moist heat (3 oz)	167
Scallops, cooked with dry heat (3 oz)	47
Tuna, light meat, canned in oil, drained	15
Egg white	0

Food	Cholesterol (mg)
Egg yolk	213
Egg substitute, frozen (¼ cup)	1
Cheddar cheese (1 oz)	30
Cottage cheese, 1% fat, (½ cup)	5
Skim milk (1 cup)	4
Low-fat milk (1%) (1 cup)	10
Whole milk (3.3% fat) (1 cup)	33
Plain yogurt, nonfat (1 cup)	4

Source: Adapted from "Step by Step, Eating to Lower Your High Blood Cholesterol," an online pamphlet from the National Institutes of Health, National Heart, Lung, and Blood Institute. (http://www.nhlbi.nih.gov/nhlbi/cardio/chol/gp/sbs-chol/tables.htm)

◆

Q: What's the story with fiber? Can it really help to lower cholesterol levels?
A: Yes. Fiber was recognized as a powerful laxative by Hippocrates in the fifth century B.C. Since then doctors have discovered that it can do a lot more than just keep you "regular." Fiber is the name given to indigestible substances found in fruits, vegetables, grains, and nuts. While fiber is an important part of a balanced diet, not *all* kinds of fiber are necessarily beneficial to your heart health. There are two main kinds, soluble and insoluble, and they are each important for different reasons. Studies suggest that soluble fiber can help lower total and LDL cholesterol. It does this in two ways. First of all, soluble fiber helps to block the absorption

of bile acids in the small intestine. What does bile have to do with cholesterol levels? Made in the liver, bile is composed of cholesterol, bilirubin (the pigment that gives stool its color), and other substances whose detergent-like action is important in breaking down and digesting food. When soluble fiber interferes with the job of bile, your body responds by drawing upon cholesterol reserves in your blood in order to manufacture more bile. The result is lower cholesterol levels. Soluble fiber is also thought to reduce blood cholesterol "at the source" by slowing its production in the liver. This type of fiber may reduce the risk of heart disease in indirect ways as well. Some studies suggest that soluble fiber may help to control blood glucose (sugar) levels and reduce the amount of insulin required by people with type 1 diabetes. As you saw in Chapter 3, people with diabetes are at high risk for heart disease but may be able to offset that risk by properly managing their condition. Good sources of soluble fiber include oat bran and oatmeal, beans such as green beans and kidney beans, peas, rice bran, barley, oranges and other citrus fruits, strawberries, and apples.

◆
Foods High in Fiber

There are good reasons to eat both kinds of fiber— and plenty of it. It is recommended that you get about 20 to 35 g of fiber each day. Most Americans consume less than half that amount. To help lower cholesterol levels, about 25% of your daily intake of fiber (about 5 to 9 g) should be soluble. Many fiber-containing foods contain both kinds of fiber but in different amounts.

Food	Serving Size	Soluble Fiber (g)	Total Fiber (g)
Apple	Unpeeled, 1 medium	2.3	3.9
Tangerine	1 medium	1.4	1.8
Plums	2 medium	1.3	2.3
Broccoli	½ cup, cooked	1.6	2.6
Kidney beans	½ cup, cooked	0.5	4.5
Pinto beans	½ cup, cooked	2.2	2.9
Oatmeal	1 cup, cooked	0.5	1.6
Whole-grain bread	1 slice	0.1	2.9

Note: While not dangerous, rapidly increasing your fiber intake to recommended levels can initially cause gas and cramping. Eat more fiber the smart way. Try adding it to your diet over a period of one or two weeks and drink an adequate amount of water (six to eight glasses) as well.

◆

Q: Does insoluble fiber lower cholesterol, too?
A: No, but it is important for other reasons. Insoluble fiber is found mainly in wheat bran and whole wheat bread, cabbage, carrots, Brussels sprouts, and cauliflower. This type of fiber helps to prevent constipation by speeding the passage of food through the colon. The colon is the tube connecting the small intestine with the anus. It is in the colon that food digested in the small intestine is further broken down and converted into stool. Insoluble fiber may also lower your risk of colon cancer, the second most common cancer in the United States, by diluting concentrations of carcinogens and helping you

to eliminate them from your body faster. (Some recent data suggest, however, that this may not be true in women.) The faster these carcinogens are out of your system, the less time they have to affect the walls of the colon.

Q: How many kinds of cholesterol are there?

A: There is really only *one* kind of cholesterol. This is an excellent question because it gives us an opportunity to clarify the way you think about cholesterol. Some people find themselves scratching their heads over the fact that doctors measure cholesterol levels in different ways. They do this not only to determine how *much* cholesterol is in your blood but also to get an idea of what your body is *doing* with that cholesterol—as you will see later in this chapter, this is where low-density lipoprotein (LDL) and high-density lipoprotein (HDL) cholesterol enter the picture. These two measurements of cholesterol are sometimes used to give you and your doctor a better picture of how your body is using cholesterol and how much of it is likely to end up in the wrong place— namely, in plaque deposits on artery walls. Total blood cholesterol is the most common measurement of blood cholesterol. There is good reason for this. Knowing your total cholesterol level—HDL cholesterol is often evaluated at the same time—is an important step in determining your risk of heart disease. (It should be noted, however, that your LDL cholesterol measurement is actually a better predictor of your risk for heart disease because of the association between high LDL levels and cardiovascular disease.) A desirable total cholesterol level is less than 200 mg/dL. A borderline-high level is between 200 and 239 mg/dL while a level of 240 mg/dL or above is considered high and can dramatically increase the likelihood of cardiovascular disease. The 38 million Americans with high cholesterol have *twice* the risk of heart disease as those whose levels are below 200 mg/dL.

Q: Can you explain how doctors measure cholesterol and what the different terms mean?
A: Doctors can measure how much cholesterol is in your blood and also test for the proteins that carry cholesterol from one place to another in your body. HDL and LDL cholesterol shed light on whether cholesterol is being deposited on your artery walls or carried to the liver where it is made into other substances or eliminated from the body altogether.

- *Cholesterol.* This waxy substance, which is classified as a steroid, is produced by your body and found in foods that come from animals. While it is necessary for good health, cholesterol is also one of the key building blocks of the plaque that sometimes develops in arteries leading to the heart and brain. Doctors recommend that you consume no more than 300 mg a day of cholesterol.
- *Total cholesterol.* This is the most common of cholesterol measurements. High cholesterol levels put you at risk for CAD because they increase the likelihood that some of this excess cholesterol will find its way onto the linings of your arteries.
- *HDL cholesterol.* When it comes to this so-called "good" cholesterol, more is better. HDL cholesterol transports less cholesterol than LDL cholesterol and carries it away from the arteries

and back to the liver where it is eliminated or transformed into other substances needed by the body.

- *LDL cholesterol.* LDL cholesterol carries most of the cholesterol in your blood. Unfortunately it has a tendency to dump its cargo of cholesterol onto the arteries, where it can accumulate and form plaque. This explains why it is referred to as "bad" cholesterol and why lower levels are better. LDL cholesterol is more important as an indicator of heart disease risk than total or HDL cholesterol.

- *VLDL (very low-density lipoprotein).* This lipoprotein primarily transports triglycerides in your blood and is discussed Chapter 6.

Q: Total cholesterol is pretty easy to understand, but what is the purpose of measuring good and bad cholesterol?
A: Measuring good or bad cholesterol is sometimes necessary to help you and your doctor understand where the cholesterol in your body is *going*. This will become clearer as we take a look at what HDL and LDL cholesterol are and how they differ. We can start with the word *lipoprotein.* Lipoproteins are complexes of proteins and cholesterol that travel through the body. Because cholesterol is a waxy substance, it does not dissolve in the blood and must travel through the body by riding "piggyback" on lipoproteins. LDL cholesterol and HDL cholesterol differ from one another in terms of the amount of cholesterol they carry and where they deposit their cholesterol cargo. LDL cholesterol carries the most cholesterol and tends to deposit it onto the lining of your arteries where it may build up and form plaque.

This explains why it is referred to as bad cholesterol. A desirable level of LDL cholesterol is less than 130 mg/dL. Cholesterol levels of 130 to 159 mg/dL are borderline high, while levels of 160 mg/dL or above mean you have a high risk of developing CAD. While an LDL cholesterol measurement is not necessary for your first cholesterol test, your doctor may recommend that you have your LDL cholesterol level checked if your total cholesterol level is high or your HDL cholesterol is low. Even a borderline total cholesterol count, when accompanied by other risk factors for CAD, may prompt your doctor to order a test for bad cholesterol because it is a better indicator of heart disease risk. HDL cholesterol is referred to as the good cholesterol because it carries its smaller cholesterol cargo (about 25% to 33% of blood cholesterol) *away* from the arteries and deposits it in the liver. HDL cholesterol removes excess cholesterol from plaque and slows its growth. Once cholesterol is transported to the liver it is passed from the body or is used to make other substances. When it comes to HDL cholesterol, a higher number actually lowers your risk of CAD. A desirable HDL cholesterol level is 46 mg/dL or higher.

◆

Do You Know Your Cholesterol Levels?

It is recommended that all adults age 20 or over have their total cholesterol levels checked at least once every five years. HDL cholesterol is often tested at the same time. Your doctor will check these levels by taking a small blood sample from your finger or hand. Fasting before cholesterol testing is unnecessary unless you are having your LDL cholesterol checked as well. If this is the case, you must avoid all food and drink for about ten hours before the test except for water, coffee, or tea—but remember to hold the cream and sugar.

	Desirable	Borderline Risk	High Risk
Total cholesterol	Less than 200 mg/dL	200 to 239 mg/dL	240 mg/dL or higher
LDL cholesterol	Less than 130 mg/dL	130 to 159 mg/dL	160 mg/dL or higher
HDL cholesterol	35 mg/dL or higher (45 mg/dL or higher for women)	Less than 35 mg/dL	Less than 35 mg/dL
LDL cholesterol/HDL cholesterol ratio	Less than 3.5 mg/dL		3.5 mg/dL or higher

Note: These are general guidelines and may not be best for you. Generally, people that have total cholesterol level less than 160 mg/dL and LDL levels less than 100 mg/dL do not develop coronary artery disease. ◆

Q: I've heard some pretty wild claims about antioxidant vitamins. Can they really protect me from heart disease? How much of these vitamins do I need to take?
A: Those are good questions. You need a quick lesson in free radicals before you can understand what antioxidant vitamins are and what they can and cannot do. In earlier

chapters of this book you learned how vital it is that your heart and other parts of the body receive a sufficient supply of oxygen. So it may seem strange to imagine that the basic process of metabolism can actually have an unhealthy effect on certain tissues, yet doctors believe this to be true. When your body's cells use oxygen to burn fat, molecular fragments of oxygen called free radicals are produced as a byproduct. Once unleashed, free radicals roam through the body causing damage to cells and to genes that regulate how cells grow—a process called oxidation. What does all this have to do with heart disease? Free radicals can damage LDL cholesterol and cause it to build up in the walls of arteries in the form of plaque. The wanton cellular destructiveness caused by free radicals may also make you more vulnerable to cancer and other diseases and even accelerate the aging process. Eliminating free radical damage is not an option since the simple act of breathing can trigger the release of these potentially destructive substances. But it is believed that antioxidants—a group of vitamins that includes vitamins E and C and beta carotene (a form of vitamin A)—may help to contain free radical damage. Some of these antioxidants are produced by the body but most are consumed through food. What doctors and the American public alike want to know is whether these vitamins can offer greater protection against heart disease and other health problems when consumed in amounts that exceed the recommended daily allowance (RDA). Although this question remains to be answered, some doctors believe that antioxidants play a role in preventing cardiovascular disease. One recent study, for example, found that women with diets high in foods containing vitamin E and beta carotene had a lower risk of heart attack and stroke. Studies of vitamin C indicate that it may help to lower blood pressure and cholesterol levels.

Q: What are some good sources of the anti-oxidant vitamins?
A: Antioxidant vitamins occur naturally in many foods. Doctors are studying the effects of higher than normal dosages of antioxidants to determine if they can prevent heart disease.

- *Vitamin E (RDA: 30 IU).* Sources of vitamin E include whole grain breads and cereals, nuts, peanut butter, and dark green, leafy vegetables such as broccoli, spinach, kale, and romaine lettuce. This vitamin is also found in vegetable oil and products derived from it such as margarine or salad dressings. Note: If you have diabetes or a heart condition or are taking high blood pressure medication, you should take vitamin E supplements only under a doctor's supervision. Vitamin E may increase the blood-thinning effects of drugs such as warfarin (Coumadin, Panwarfin, or Sofarin) or aspirin. Also, if you are considering taking vitamin E as a preventive measure, consult your doctor first; some studies have shown that (depending on dose) vitamin E alone may cause blood thinning.

- *Vitamin C (RDA: 60 mg).* Most of us already know that oranges and other citrus fruits are excellent sources of vitamin C (one 8-ounce glass of orange juice, for example, supplies 100% of the vitamin C you need each day). But did you know that other foods rich in vitamin C include sweet peppers, broccoli, potatoes, strawberries, and other berries? If you plan to take vitamin C supplements, make sure that you drink plenty of water, as large doses of vitamin C can increase your risk of kidney stones.

- *Beta carotene (no RDA).* Beta carotene is found
  in yellow or orange vegetables such as carrots,
  pumpkins, winter squash, and sweet potatoes. It
  is contained in fruits of that color such as can-
  taloupe and peaches. Dark green, leafy vegetables are also good sources of beta carotene.
  Studies are still underway to determine if beta
  carotene has preventive effects for heart disease.
  If you plan to take beta carotene supplements,
  consult your doctor first.

**Q: Is there any harm in taking high doses of
antioxidant vitamins?**

A: There could be. While some studies of antioxidant
vitamins are intriguing, most national health organizations do not recommend exceeding the RDA of these
vitamins for the time being. We simply do not have
enough reliable answers at this point. How exactly do
antioxidants produce their healthy effects? Until doctors
understand the mechanism of action behind antioxidants
they are hesitant to endorse their preventive powers. Are
antioxidants really responsible for the disease-fighting
effects of antioxidant-rich fruits and vegetables or do
these plants contain other, as yet unidentified substances
that help to prevent illness? What are the long-term side
effects of taking high dosages of these vitamins? Until
these questions are answered, most doctors recommend
that you get your RDA of antioxidants by eating three to
five servings of vegetables and two to four servings of
fruit each day. Supplements should be considered when
you are unable to get the RDA of these vitamins through
your diet. If you are cutting back on calories as part of a
weight-loss program or do not eat enough fruits and vegetables for any reason, talk to your doctor or a registered
dietitian about taking a multivitamin supplement.

Q: Does drinking alcohol help to prevent heart disease?

A: It appears that it does but only in small amounts. The use of alcohol in preventing heart disease is a matter of controversy in the medical community. This explains why you do not hear doctors trumpeting the virtues of wine and beer with unbridled enthusiasm. The facts are these: Studies suggest that people who drink moderate amounts of alcohol—one or two drinks a day for men and one drink daily for women—have lower rates of heart disease than nondrinkers. The one or two drinks of liquor a day (one drink is 12 ounces of beer or 4 ounces of wine) appear to offer a partially protective effect through an increase in HDL cholesterol levels.

Many doctors and national health organizations tend to take a conservative view of alcohol use not because they are making a moral stand but because they are all too aware of the many health problems associated with drinking. Alcohol can contribute to high blood pressure and obesity and raise blood triglyceride levels. It can also increase your risk of alcoholism, osteoporosis (this is of particular concern for postmenopausal women), and stroke. For a complex variety of reasons that we do not fully understand, some people are able to drink in moderation while others develop a dependency on alcohol. Even small amounts of alcohol may put certain people at risk for serious medical conditions. According to a recent study, one drink of alcohol a day may raise a woman's risk of dying of breast cancer by 11%. As you can see, there are a number of factors to consider when it comes to alcohol and heart disease risk. Your doctor can help you determine the potential benefits and risks of moderate drinking depending on the presence of existing medical conditions such as osteoporosis as well as your specific health concerns. For example, if you are a post-menopausal women in good cardiovascular health but you are at risk for osteoporosis or breast cancer, drinking alcohol even in moderation may not be the right choice for you. Note: People on aspirin therapy should avoid alcohol.

◆

Factors That Affect Your Cholesterol Levels

A number of factors can influence your cholesterol levels—from dietary fats and exercise to your age and gender.

- *Food and drink.* Saturated fat can raise your cholesterol levels more than the cholesterol you get from food. Unsaturated fats such as polyunsaturated fat and monounsaturated fat may help to lower cholesterol levels, although some studies suggest that polyunsaturated fat may not actually lower levels. Eating too much of most foods can lead to obesity and excess blood fats. As you have seen earlier in this chapter, other things in your diet such as fiber, antioxidant vitamins, and even alcohol (in moderation) can influence your blood cholesterol as well. See Chapter 5 for more information on saturated and other fats in your diet.
- *Exercise.* Aerobic exercise may increase levels of heart-healthy HDL cholesterol.
- *Weight.* Being obese or overweight puts a strain on the heart and can lower good cholesterol levels. See Chapter 5 for more information on obesity.
- *Heredity.* While genes are not necessarily destiny, they may affect how your body produces and uses cholesterol. If you are susceptible to high cholesterol levels, it is even more important to

eliminate or control your other risk factors for high cholesterol.

* *Age.* Blood cholesterol levels tend to rise as we age. Women generally have lower cholesterol levels than men at younger ages, but after menopause more women than men have excess cholesterol in their blood.

Source: From the National Heart, Lung, and Blood Institute (http://www.nhlbi.nih.gov). ◆

What Are Triglycerides?

Nicole, age 14, is an active girl who is slightly overweight for her age. At her last checkup, a cholesterol screening was done and her parents were surprised to find that their daughter had an elevated cholesterol level. Her tests also revealed elevated low-density lipoprotein (LDL) cholesterol and triglyceride levels. Her high-density lipoprotein (HDL) cholesterol level was fine, though a little on the low side.

Nicole's parents had an abundance of questions for the pediatrician, including "What does this mean for Nicole's health?" "Should we be controlling her cholesterol level at this age?" "Won't this mean cutting back on needed calcium products such as milk and cheese?" "Will a low-fat diet affect our daughter's growth?"

The pediatrician reviewed Nicole's diet with her parents and discussed with them the meaning of the laboratory findings. The doctor also explained, to their surprise, that fatty deposits can begin to develop in the coronary arteries during childhood and continue to progress for decades. Obesity, even when it occurs in youth, can increase the risk of developing heart disease later in life. As is often the case, weight problems ran in Nicole's family.

Nicole's diet, while not completely unhealthy, included too many foods high in saturated fat. Although her dinners at home with her parents were quite nutritious (broiled chicken, fish, rice, and pasta were staples), her school lunch selections and after-school snacking habits were not as healthy. For lunch at school she always chose whole instead of low-fat milk and often selected pizza, fried fish, french fries, and tacos. Her after-school snacks with friends and at home included too many high-fat foods such as doughnuts, potato chips, and ice cream.

Nicole's doctor explained that dietary changes could help her to lose weight and lower her cholesterol and triglyceride levels without sacrificing the calcium, protein, and other nutrients she needed for healthy growth. Nicole was told how to make better food selections at lunchtime and after school. She was put on a low-fat, low-cholesterol diet that included drinking skim milk (instead of whole milk), limiting her intake of pizza to one slice a week, avoiding fried foods, and substituting healthier snacks—pretzels, butterless popcorn, fruit, or a scoop of low-fat yogurt—for her usual high-fat treats. Her parents also started buying natural peanut butter that had no hydrogenated fats added, as peanut butter was a favorite of their daughter's. They limited her intake to two peanut butter sandwiches a week. Nicole was also told that the occasional cookie or doughnut would not ruin her diet, *but that an apple, banana, or other fruit would be a better choice.*

After six months on her new diet, Nicole noticed with pleasure that her clothes were fitting better and both she and her parents were pleased to find that her cholesterol and triglyceride levels were quite close to normal. Nicole did not find the changes in her diet that difficult and she found that she enjoyed her new, healthier food choices just as much as the foods she used to eat. Nicole's pediatrician praised her success and told her that her new dietary habits were important in order to live a healthy adult life and lower her risk of heart disease in the future.

From no-fat potato chips and cholesterol-lowering olive oil to trans fatty acids, health-savvy Americans have developed a keen interest in fat. What exactly *are* fats and why do they play such an important role in our heart health? Most of the fats in our food and our bodies are triglycerides. You already know more about triglycerides than you think. They are another name for almost everything that we consider "fat." Just consider where they are found.

- *Your food.* Triglycerides are the fats in your food. They include the dietary fats in everything from hot fudge sundaes and vegetable oil to french fries and swordfish. The fats you may know as saturated or polyunsaturated fat, for example, are triglycerides. Is cholesterol a triglyceride? No. In fact, cholesterol is not even a fat. This waxy substance is classified as a steroid.
- *Your waistline.* Triglycerides are also the way that fat is stored in your body. Triglycerides are responsible for "the love handles" and those few extra pounds that some of us gain after the holidays. They are what you feel between your fingers when you squeeze the fat in your hip or thigh.

• *Your blood.* Like cholesterol, triglycerides also flow through the bloodstream. Blood triglyceride levels are sometimes measured to help determine heart disease risk.

Though many Americans have come to identify fat as the enemy, it is important to remember that triglycerides are necessary for good health. Fats are used by the body as a source of energy. When stored by the body, triglycerides help to protect and insulate internal organs and cushion the blow of a fall. So how do triglycerides affect our risk of heart disease? The answer depends largely on whether we are referring to the fats in our diet or our blood. This chapter is devoted to an explanation of the triglycerides in our food. These dietary fats can have a profound influence on our cholesterol levels and increase our risk of gaining extra weight or becoming obese. A diet high in fat is the main cause of high cholesterol levels and plaque buildup in the arteries. Dietary fats also affect triglyceride levels in our blood. The meaning and significance of blood triglyceride levels are the subject Chapters 6 and 7.

Q: What are triglycerides made of?
A: You can think of triglycerides as the way that nature "packages" most of the fats in your food and in your body. Triglycerides are composed of even smaller units of fat (called fatty acids) attached to a chemical base of glycerol. Fatty acids are known as the building blocks of fat. Most of the dietary fats discussed in this chapter are a mixture of three different kinds of fatty acids. A fatty acid is described as saturated, polyunsaturated, or monounsaturated depending on how much of the element hydrogen it contains. Saturated fatty acids contain the most hydrogen and are considered the most unhealthy. The polyunsaturated variety contain the least hydrogen

and monounsaturated fatty acids fall somewhere in between. Though most dietary fats are actually *mixtures* of all three fatty acids in different amounts, we usually describe a fat as being one or the other based on the predominance of a particular fatty acid. For example, olive oil is classified as a monounsaturated fat because it contains more fatty acids of that type than any other. If this all sounds a little confusing, do not worry. It is not crucial that you understand the relationship between fatty acids, glycerol molecules, and the hydrogen content of fat. The main thing is to understand the differences between healthy and unhealthy fats in your diet. This chapter is your guide to those fats and will help you to identify which foods contain which kind of fat.

Q: What is saturated fat and how does it affect my cholesterol levels?

A: We call fat "saturated" when it contains a high proportion of saturated fatty acids. Along with the cholesterol you get from food, saturated fat can raise your blood cholesterol levels more than anything else in your diet. Saturated fats raise your blood cholesterol levels by slowing down the removal of "bad" LDL cholesterol. Therefore, even if your diet is low in cholesterol, your blood cholesterol levels may be high if your diet contains a large amount of saturated fat. This type of fat is found in high amounts in many of the foods that Americans eat on a regular basis. Most of these foods come from animals. Examples of foods containing saturated fat include beef, pork, veal, poultry, butter, cream, milk, and cheese. These foods also contain cholesterol so they can raise your blood cholesterol levels in two ways at the same time. In addition to meat and dairy products, certain oils derived from plants also contain high amounts of saturated fat. These include coconut oil, palm kernel oil, and palm oil (known collectively as tropical oils). These oils generally cost less than their healthier counterparts, which explains why tropical oils are frequently used by companies that manufacture processed foods, including popular high-fat snacks such as potato chips. Because saturated fat is found in so many of the foods we eat, it is important to limit your intake of meat and dairy products and read food labels in order to avoid products high in this type of fat. To help maintain healthy cholesterol levels, limit your intake of saturated fat to 10% of your total calories (these guidelines apply to adults as well as to children over age two). If you consume 2,000 calories a day, for example, your saturated fat calories should not equal more than 200, which is the equivalent of about 22g of fat, because each gram of fat contains about 9 calories. People with CAD should consume even less saturated fat.

◆

America's Fast-Food Fix: A Quick Source of Fat and Cholesterol

Much of the fat and cholesterol in the American diet is hidden in its fast food. It is difficult to gauge the fat content of these foods because they do not always come with the "Nutrition Facts" labels found on products at your grocery store, although several fast-food chains—such as McDonald's— now provide nutrition information for their products. The chart below lists the saturated fat, cholesterol, and total fat content of some common fast-food items. It is recommended that you limit the total fat in your diet to no more than 30% of your total calories. It is important to note that serving sizes may vary among different fast-food chains.

Product	Saturated Fat (g)	Cholesterol (mg)	Total Fat (g)
Cheese pizza (¹/₈ of 12-in. pizza)	1.5	9	3.2
Chili con carne (1 cup)	3.4	133	8.3
Roast beef sandwich, plain	3.6	52	13.8
Hamburger, lower fat, plain	4.0	60	10.0
Hamburger, plain	4.1	36	11.8
Hot dog	5.1	44	14.5
Fish sandwich, with tartar sauce	5.2	55	22.8
Chicken, boneless pieces, breaded and fried (6 pieces)	5.5	62	17.7
Taco salad with chili (1¹/₂ cup)	6.0	4	13.1
Cheeseburger, single patty, plain	6.5	50	15.2
Burrito with beans and cheese (2 burritos)	6.8	27	11.7

Product	Saturated Fat (g)	Cholesterol (mg)	Total Fat (g)
Submarine sandwich (hero) with cold cuts	6.8	35	18.6
Chicken fillet sandwich, plain	8.5	60	29.5
Baked potato with cheese sauce and chili	13.0	31	21.9
Cheeseburger, large double patty	17.7	141	44.0
French fries, regular size order	3.8	0	12.0
Egg-and-bacon biscuit (1 biscuit)	9.9	353	31.1
Egg, bacon, and cheese biscuit (1 biscuit)	11.4	261	31.4
Chocolate shake (10 oz.)	6.5	37	10.5

Source: Adapted from "Step by Step, Eating to Lower Your High Blood Cholesterol," an online pamphlet from the National Institutes of Health, National Heart, Lung, and Blood Institute (http://www.nhlbi.nih.gov/nhlbi/cardio/chol/gp/sbs-chol/fastfood.htm).

◆

Q: Is it true that some fats can actually lower my cholesterol levels?

A: Some doctors think so, but at the moment we do not have a simple answer to this question. All doctors agree that saturated fat is the worst type of fat and that too much of any fat in your diet is unhealthy. But there is no consensus in the medical community as to the effect that unsaturated fats, such as monounsaturated and polyunsaturated fat, have on cholesterol levels. Let us first take a look at monounsaturated fat. It is found in olive, canola, and peanut oils as well as in avocados. Some experts believe that monounsaturated fat can help to reduce your LDL blood cholesterol levels without altering your HDL. Other research suggests that this type of fat has a "neutral" effect, neither increasing or lowering cholesterol levels.

So what about the other unsaturated fat? Doctors are even less certain about the effects of polyunsaturated fat on cholesterol levels. This fat is found in many cooking oils and in margarine. It is in sunflower and sesame seeds, soybeans, corn, certain nuts, and in the oils made from these plants. Some studies indicate that polyunsaturated fat is something of a double-edged sword in regard to its effect on cholesterol levels, helping to reduce LDL but also lowering heart-healthy HDL. But other data suggest that polyunsaturated fat may actually raise LDL.

What is the bottom line concerning these so-called healthy fats? When it comes to fat in your diet, you should always choose unsaturated fat instead of saturated fat. Like every other aspect of your diet, consuming monounsaturated and polyunsaturated fat in moderation is the key. It is recommended that you limit your intake of polyunsaturated fat to 10% of your total calories and your intake of monounsaturated fat to 10 to 15% of your total calories.

Q: What about other kinds of fat? Are they all harmful?

A: There are many kinds of fats, and all of them are not created equal. The different triglycerides in your diet affect cholesterol levels and other aspects of your health in different ways. Dietary fats also influence your blood triglyceride levels. Some important triglycerides include the following:

- *Saturated fat.* This type of fat can raise your cholesterol levels more than any other part of your diet—even more than the cholesterol that you get from food. This hydrogen-rich fat is considered the worst for your health. See page 86 for more information on saturated fat.
- *Monounsaturated fat.* Some doctors believe that this unsaturated fat can lower your LDL cholesterol levels without reducing your good cholesterol. Other research suggests that monounsaturated fat may be "neutral" when it comes to cholesterol levels. See page 90 for more information on monounsaturated fat.
- *Polyunsaturated fat.* Some studies indicate that polyunsaturated fat is something of a double-edged sword in regard to its effect on cholesterol levels, helping to reduce LDL but also lowering heart-healthy HDL. But other data suggest that polyunsaturated may actually raise LDL. See page 90 for more information on polyunsaturated fat.
- *Trans fatty acids.* This special breed of fatty acid occurs in small amounts in meat and dairy products. Americans consume most of it in margarine and other foods made from hydrogenated oil. Trans fatty acids are not quite as unhealthy as sat-

urated fatty acids but they can raise your cholesterol levels. See page 94 for more information on
trans fatty acids.

- *Essential fatty acids.* There are two essential
  fatty acids that cannot be produced by the body
  and must be consumed through the diet. Techni-
  cally a part of the polyunsaturated fat family,
  these fats are important for a variety of reasons.
  Your body uses them to maintain the structural
  integrity of cell membranes and to make hor-
  monelike substances called eicosanoids. These
  odd-sounding substances can help to improve
  your HDL and LDL cholesterol ratio. They also
  play a role in regulating blood pressure and circulation, preventing blood clots, and keeping the
  immune system strong. Omega-3, found primarily in fish, is also present in green leafy vegetables, nuts, and soybeans. See later in this chapter
  for more information about omega-3 and its role
  in your cardiovascular health. See page 99 for
  more information on omega-3. Omega-6 is a fatty
  acid found in fish, green leafy vegetables, grains,
  and seeds. Vegetable oils and meats also contain a
  small amount of omega-6.

**Q: What about that new fake fat they put in
potato chips? Is that for real? What effect does
it have on my health?**
A: It is known as olestra and it is not exactly a "fake fat."
After being tested in over 100 studies involving 20,000
people, this fat replacer was approved by the FDA for use
in such snack products as potato and tortilla chips and
crackers. Olestra is a response by the food industry to the
American public's demand for lower-fat foods that taste
like "the real thing." Many consumers and doctors alike

have hailed olestra as a success. Until Americans unlearn their taste for fatty foods, olestra can be a great way to enjoy an *occasional* snack food (for example, a bag of potato chips) without consuming the saturated fat that usually goes with it. Food manufacturers use olestra in place of other fats in order to create a fat-free or low-fat product with the same texture and taste of foods fried in regular oil.

Olestra is basically a fat that has been disguised so well that your body, which is designed to process the fats that occur in nature, does not "recognize" olestra as fat. Normally fats are broken down by your body during digestion and then absorbed. While it may taste like fat on your tongue, olestra is an unknown quantity as far as your intestines are concerned. Not knowing how to break it down, your body gives olestra a "green light" to pass through the body without being properly absorbed. But just because products made with olestra are often fat-free does not mean you should eat them in excess. These snack foods do not contain adequate amounts of the vitamins, minerals, and other nutrients we need for good health. Remember: Fruits, vegetables, and grains *are* rich in these nutrients while also being low in saturated fat and calories. Products made from olestra make the most sense as an occasional replacement for nature's "snack foods."

Because olestra mimics insoluble fiber in its ability to pass through the bowel unchanged, some people who eat products made with olestra experience the sort of gastrointestinal (GI) effects associated with high-fiber foods. These effects include gas, cramping, and softer stools. Not everyone experiences the GI effects associated with olestra. Of more concern is the suggestion that olestra may actually block the body's absorption of important vitamins including vitamins A, D, E, and K. This can happen when foods containing these vitamins are eaten around the same time as olestra. To help compensate for this, food companies usually add extra amounts of these vitamins to snack foods made with the fat replacer.

Q: Why are doctors so concerned about our consumption of trans fatty acids?

A: Trans fatty acids are a special breed of fatty acid. They resemble saturated fatty acids but do not contain quite as much hydrogen. Until a few decades ago, trans fatty acids were found only in meat and dairy products (in small amounts). Due to a manufacturing process known as hydrogenation, these unhealthy fatty acids are now contained in a number of processed foods. Hydrogenation involves bombarding heart-healthy polyunsaturated fatty acids (such as those found in vegetable oil) with hydrogen ions in order to enhance the shelf life of a product or thicken its consistency. Trans fatty acids are not quite as unhealthy as saturated fatty acids but they can worsen your cholesterol levels in three ways. They tend to raise total and LDL cholesterol levels while lowering HDL cholesterol. So why use hydrogenation in the first place? Ironically, the answer to this question involves an attempt by food manufacturers to use healthier oils in response to pressure from national health organizations. Here is the rub: Vegetable oils consisting of polyunsaturated fatty acids spoil faster than unhealthy oils and tend to be softer. In order to thicken healthy oils and create products such as margarine sticks, hydrogenation is used. In order to steer clear of trans fatty acids, choose a margarine in tub or liquid form. The more "solid" a margarine is, the greater the likelihood that it is hydrogenated. You should also avoid processed foods that list "hydrogenated" or "partially hydrogenated" oil as an ingredient. About 80% to 90% of the trans fatty acids in the American diet come from hydrogenated vegetable oil.

Q: What is obesity and how does it affect my risk of heart disease?

A: Obesity is an excess of body fat that equals 20% or more of your "ideal" weight. This is the amount that you are expected to weigh based on variables such as your gender and height. Three out of four Americans are overweight to some degree and about 34 million are considered obese. Being overweight can have serious consequences on our cardiovascular health. The system composed of your heart and blood vessels operates most efficiently when your weight falls within a certain range. Carrying around extra pounds puts unnecessary strain on the heart, making it work harder to do the same job. Genetic predisposition plays a major role in the storage of excess fat. Eating a diet high in fat and calories and not getting enough exercise are also important factors in weight gain, as are underlying medical conditions such as hypothyroidism, Cushing's syndrome, and Turner's syndrome. Studies suggest that the *location* of extra body fat—and not just the *amount*—can increase the risk of developing a variety of weight-related health problems. Too much fat in the abdomen, for example, is considered more unhealthy than storing extra pounds in the hips and thighs. Having a "spare tire" in the midsection may increase your risk of premature heart disease, diabetes, hypertension, and cancer.

There are no short cuts to weight loss. Eating a low-fat, low-calorie diet and getting regular aerobic exercise are the safest and most effective ways to reach your weight goals. When it comes to trimming the fat, a little can mean a lot. Losing just 5 to 10 pounds, for example, can help to improve your cholesterol levels if you are already overweight. Over-the-counter (OTC) and prescription medications are sometimes used in the short term to aid weight loss. Some of these medications are designed to curb the appetite while others boost levels of serotonin in the brain. In proper amounts this hormone helps to control appetite and also produces a sense of emotional well-being. Always talk to your doctor before using an OTC or prescription medication for weight reduction. Some of these drugs can have unwanted and even dangerous side effects. Newer agents on the horizon may be capable of aiding in weight loss without the risks associated with currently available medications.

◆

Avoid Seesaw Dieting—Exercise!

When it comes to losing weight, there is no substitute for eating a low-fat, nutritious diet and getting plenty of exercise. Do not be fooled by weight-loss programs or fad diets that promise to help you shed pounds overnight. The "dieting" trap can often lead to a vicious and emotionally destructive cycle in which you lose weight in the short term and gain it back in weeks or months. Quick weight-loss schemes can actually slow your metabolism and lead to low self-esteem, dangerous eating disorders, and depression. Some doctors even believe that seesaw dieting can increase your risk of heart disease and other health problems in the long run. Exercise is an important part of any serious commitment to losing weight. Approach weight loss the smart way by making gradual changes in your lifestyle. A safe rate of weight loss is generally considered $1/2$ to 1 pound a week. A variety of activities can burn calories and help you to maintain an ideal weight—from gardening and jogging to skiing down mountain slopes.

Average calories expended in an hour*

Activity	120 to 130 lb person	170 to 180 lb person
Aerobic dancing	290-575	400-800
Backpacking	290-630	400-880
Badminton	230-515	320-720
Basketball		
Game	400-690	560-960
Nongame	170-515	240-720
Bicycling		
Outdoor	170-800	240-1,120
Stationary	85-800	120-1,120
Bowling	115-170	160-240
Dancing	115-400	160-560
Gardening	115-400	160-560
Golfing (walking, carrying or pulling bags)	115-400	160-560
Handball	170-690	640-960
Hiking	170-690	240-960
Jogging		
5 mph (12 min/mile)	460	640
6 mph (10 min/mile)	575	800
Racquetball	345-690	480-960

*The range of calories listed here depends on how vigorously the activity is performed. The ranges are from lowest to highest intensity.

Activity	120 to 130 lb person	170 to 180 lb person
Running		
7 mph (9 min/mile)	690	960
8 mph (7.5 min/mile)	745	1,040
10 mph (6 min/mile)	860	1,200
Scuba diving	290-690	400-800
Skating, ice or roller	230-460	320-640
Skiing		
Cross-country	290-800	400-1,120
Downhill	170-460	240-640
Soccer	290-690	400-960
Squash	345-690	480-960
Stair-climbing	230-460	320-640
Swimming	230-690	320-900
Tennis	230-515	320-720
Volleyball	170-400	240-560
Walking		
2 mph (30 min/mile)	150	210
3 mph (20 min/mile)	200	275
4 mph (15 min/mile)	250	340

Source: By permission of the Mayo Foundation.

Q: Can eating fish help to prevent heart disease?
A: It appears that it can. Doctors speculate that the omega-3 fatty acids in fish are what makes it healthy for the heart. The role of fish in heart-disease prevention first came up a few decades ago when doctors were studying Inuit (Eskimos) in Greenland. These Inuits presented something of a puzzle to researchers. They ate diets high in fat and yet had a low rate of heart attack. The answer appeared to lie in the large amount of fish and whale meat that these Inuits consumed on a daily basis. Since then doctors have intensified their study of omega-fatty acids and determined that they have several benefits on your health when eaten regularly. For one thing, these fatty acids appear to lower triglyceride levels in your blood. As you will see in Chapter 6, blood triglyceride levels are sometimes a risk factor for coronary artery disease (CAD). If you have very high blood triglyceride levels, your doctor may even recommend fish oil supplements along with your medication. Being "natural" blood thinners, omega-3 fatty acids may also reduce the risk of the sort of blood clot that can lead to a heart attack or stroke. Studies also suggest that omega-3 fatty acids may lower blood pressure.

Salmon, herring, and mackerel are particularly good sources of omega-3 fatty acids, which are also found in lesser amounts in green leafy vegetables, nuts, and soybeans. It is recommended that you eat at least two meals of fish every week for possible heart benefits. Eating more than that may not increase the protective effect and may even expose you to unhealthy levels of mercury, a toxin sometimes present in fish in small amounts. Are fish oil capsules an option? They may be if you are unable to eat two meals of fish each week, but they are not recommended for several reasons. First of all, doctors are not certain exactly *why* eating fish is so good for

your health. Is it the omega-3 fatty acids alone that provide protection from cardiovascular disease or a combination of these and other substances contained in fish?
Some doctors speculate that adding fish to your diet may
reduce your risk of heart disease because of what it does
not contain—namely, the high amounts of saturated fat
present in meat. The answer may even be "all of the
above." Note: If you are on aspirin therapy or are taking
the medication warfarin (Coumadin, Panwarfin, or
Sofarin), talk to your doctor before taking fish oil supplements. They may affect the blood-thinning effects of
these drugs.

◆

The Mediterranean Diet Study:
A Fish Story

Results from the Lyon Diet Heart Study suggest
that eating a Mediterranean-style diet rich in
omega-3 fatty acids may greatly reduce the risk of
a second heart attack. The study, which was conducted in France and reported in the medical journal *Circulation* in early 1999, involved more than
400 men and women who had already suffered
heart attacks. About half this number ate a
Mediterranean diet while the other half ate a
higher-fat, Western-style diet that was lower in
omega-3 fatty acids. The Mediterranean diet,
which is similar to that eaten by people who live
near the Mediterranean Sea, consists largely of
fruits, vegetables, fish, cereals, and beans. People
in the Lyon Diet Heart Study who ate a Mediterranean diet for almost four years were 50% to 70%
less likely to suffer another heart attack or other
cardiovascular problems (such as stroke or blood
clots) when compared to the Western-diet (control)

group. Men and women in both groups were similar in terms of their risk factors for heart disease—body fat, blood cholesterol levels, and blood pressure were comparable between the two groups at the start of the study. People on the Western-style diet consumed about 34% of calories from fat, and their intake of saturated fat was about 12% of total calories. The Mediterranean-diet group got about 30% of calories from fat, and their intake of saturated fat was 8% of total calories. People in the latter group had higher blood levels of omega-3 fatty acids at the conclusion of the study, suggesting that this type of polyunsaturated fat may offer some measure of protection against cardiovascular disease.

◆

Q: I was always taught that it was okay for kids to eat whatever they want—that their systems can "handle it." After having a heart attack and being diagnosed with CAD, I'm starting to wonder if I'm doing enough to make sure that this never happens to my kids. Is there anything I can do to help them avoid these sorts of problems as adults?

A: Many doctors would say yes. If we start making changes in our diet and lifestyle during youth, we may be able to delay or help prevent some of the health problems associated with aging—from heart disease and osteoporosis to certain kinds of cancer. It is true that most cases of CAD are diagnosed after midlife. But the narrowing and hardening of the arteries that we refer to as atherosclerosis actually begins to develop in childhood or young adulthood—and this is a great time to start doing something about it. The dietary fats that our children consume are a major reason for the development of plaque in their arteries. But some parents, as well as some doctors and nutritionists, discourage low-fat diets for children because of myths that these diets can impede growth or are insufficient in the vitamins and minerals necessary for proper development. A 1998 article published in the *American Journal of Cardiology* emphasizes the importance of teaching our children how to eat a diet low in unhealthy fats and rich in plant-based foods in order to prevent heart disease later in life. This article describes 12 myths that persist in the medical community and in the minds of the American public. Some of these myths* are explained below.

- *Myth: Controlling cholesterol can wait.* A diet high in fat is one of the major reasons that there are 50 million children in the United States with elevated cholesterol levels. About 70% of children have fatty deposits in their coronary arteries by age 12, and the early stages of CAD can be seen in almost every young adult by age 21.
- *Myth: Controlling obesity can wait.* An obese child is twice as likely to die of heart disease before age 70 as peers who do not have a weight problem. This risk does not decrease if the child loses weight later in life, which emphasizes the need to maintain an ideal weight even in youth. If you are obese, there is a 40% chance that your child will become obese as well. This risk jumps

*Reprinted from *American Journal of Cardiology*, Vol. 82, Attwood CR. "Low-fat diets for children: Practicality and Safety," pp 77-79, 1998, with permission from Excerpta Medica Inc.

to 80% if both parents have a weight problem. Genes are the main reason that obesity tends to run in families. But transmitting bad eating habits from parent to child is thought to play an important role as well. As you have seen earlier in this chapter, obesity is a risk factor for heart disease and other health problems such as high blood pressure and diabetes.

• *Myth: Children's diets are getting better.* Wrong! Too many of our children rely on readily available snack foods and fast food for their calories. Due to our busy schedules, we often are not with them to help guide their dietary decision-making. Restaurant chains compete with each other to make larger and larger hamburgers. The biggest name in fast food, McDonald's, even discontinued their McLean Deluxe several years ago because sales of the lower-fat burger were poor. The trend is in the opposite direction—bigger and fattier burgers.

• *Myth: Low-fat diets lack vitamins and minerals.* Even a vegetarian diet can provide adequate vitamins and minerals when a proper number of calories are eaten. Providing vitamin B_{12} via a multivitamin, B_{12}-fortified cereal, or meat substitutes should be considered for children whose diets contain no animal products.

• *Myth: Low-fat diets retard growth.* Earlier studies had indicated that low-fat diets may retard growth in children. Most doctors no longer believe this to be true. Children age two or older with diets low in fat can achieve normal growth, and recent research suggests that even children on supervised vegetarian diets grow at proper rates. Note: It is not recommended that children younger than age two be placed on low-fat diets.

- *Myth: Children will not eat a plant-based diet.* As most parents know, children are creatures of habit. It is true that they may not show initial enthusiasm for changes in their diets. This is because healthier foods are often unfamiliar to them. Try taking your child grocery shopping. Steer clear of steaks and chops and spend some time in the produce section. Talk to them about different vegetables, the nutrients they contain, and the different ways they can be prepared. Simply habituating your child to the *idea* of a diet rich in plant foods is half the battle because it usually requires "unlearning" some unhealthy eating habits. Parents also need to explain the importance of whole grains and fiber.

What can parents do to teach their kids the importance of cardiovascular health? For one thing, do not buy into myths such as those outlined above. Make an effort to limit the amount of fat in your child's diet. You can refer to the guidelines for dietary fat intake described earlier in this chapter for specifics on how much saturated fat should be a part of total calorie consumption. Talk to your doctor, pediatrician, or a registered dietician about trimming the fat from your child's diet safely—especially if you intend to eliminate animal products such as meat or milk.

◆

The Food Guide Pyramid: Helping You and Your Family Make Smart Dietary Choices

Eating right is a lot easier than you may think. The U.S. Department of Agriculture (USDA) has provided recommendations for healthy eating called the Food Guide Pyramid. Think of it as a new and improved version of the Four Food Groups that you learned about while growing up. By following these general dietary guidelines, you and other members of your family two years of age or older can limit the saturated fat, cholesterol, and sodium in your diet while getting the nutrients you need for good health—including heart-healthy antioxidant vitamins. The basic idea is apparent at a glance: Eat more grains, fruits, and vegetables and cut back on your consumption of meat, dairy products, and fat. The USDA recommends that you eat at least the lowest numbers of servings from each of the groups listed below in order to get proper amounts of vitamins, minerals, carbohydrates, and protein.

- *Bread, cereal, rice, and pasta.* Eat 6 to 11 servings a day. Examples: A serving is one slice of bread, 1 ounce of cereal, or ½ cup of cooked cereal, rice, or pasta.
- *Vegetables.* Eat 3 to 5 servings a day. Examples: A serving is 1 cup of raw, leafy vegetables; ½ cup of other vegetables, cooked or chopped raw; or ¾ cup of vegetable juice.
- *Fruit.* Eat 2 to 4 servings a day. Examples: A serving is one medium apple, banana, or orange;

$^1/_2$ cup of chopped, cooked, or canned fruit; or $^3/_4$ cup of fruit juice.

- *Meat, poultry, fish, dry beans, eggs, and nuts.* Eat 2 to 3 servings a day. Examples: A serving is 2 to 3 ounces of cooked lean meat, poultry, or fish; $^1/_2$ cup of cooked dry beans or one egg counts as 1 ounce of lean meat; 2 tablespoons of peanut butter or $^1/_3$ cup of nuts count as 1 ounce of meat.
- *Milk, yogurt, and cheese.* Eat 2 to 3 servings a day. Examples: A serving is 1 cup of milk or yogurt, $1^1/_2$ ounces of natural cheese, or 2 ounces of processed cheese.
- *Fats, oils, and sweets.* Use sparingly.

Source: The USDA's Food Guide Pyramid: A Guide to Daily Food Choices. Online source is http://www.nal.usda.gov:8001/py/pmap.htm.

◆

The USDA's Food Guide Pyramid: A guide to daily food choices.

Source: U.S. Department of Agriculture. From Stolar, Mark and Annussek, Greg A. *Evista®* (*raloxifene*). Avon WholeCare, New York, copyright ©1999, CMD Publishing.

6

How Your Body Uses Triglycerides

QUICK FACT

◆

*Recent changes in weight can
artificially elevate or lower your
triglyceride level.*

Andrea, age 32, had not had her cholesterol and triglyceride levels checked in about five years. The last time she had her cholesterol checked, her levels were within normal limits. When I recently tested her, the LDL or "bad" cholesterol and triglycerides were elevated, falling in the borderline-high range. Andrea was surprised; she had not thought her cholesterol level and triglycerides would ever be a problem because she did not usually eat many high-fat foods.

I asked Andrea to tell me about her lifestyle. She explained that she had put on some weight within the last three months (approximately 10 pounds), which put her in the slightly overweight range. Andrea attributed her weight gain to her new job. Previously, she had worked as a foreign correspondent, which kept her on the go. But 4 *months ago she had begun her current position—working as an editor for a magazine, a more sedentary job. Andrea also described her new job as more stressful, and explained that she began overeating to cope with her stress. On especially bad days at work, she did not pay attention to how much food she was eating, and would often snack on high-calorie, low-fat snacks all day. When she came home she was tired, and she sometimes would eat double portions. The combination of sedentary lifestyle, stress, and overeating had conspired to cause her subsequent weight gain.*

I explained to Andrea that a sudden weight gain could produce an artificially high test result, an inaccurate reading of triglycerides. I explained to Andrea that the more food she consumed, the higher her triglyceride levels could potentially be. She would need to come for a retest as soon as her weight had stabilized for a few months. In the meantime I suggested that she consider gradually modifying her diet by choosing nutritious, low-fat foods more consistently and eating smaller portions, as well as adopting an exercise regimen that would enable her to lower her LDL cholesterol and raise her HDL cholesterol. I pointed out to her that an exercise program would have an added psychological benefit—it would help to keep her stress level down. She agreed to adopt a new lifestyle regimen and to come for a retest in a few months when her weight had stabilized.

Andrea came to see me five months later. Her cholesterol and triglycerides were both within normal limits. Andrea continued to adhere to her new exercise and lifestyle regimen, keeping her focus on losing excess weight gradually.

Doctors mainly rely on cholesterol measurements to evaluate the likelihood of plaque buildup in arteries leading to the heart or brain. Not only do we measure the total amount of cholesterol but we can also evaluate HDL and LDL cholesterol. By looking at HDL and particularly LDL, we get a better picture of how the body is using cholesterol and whether it and other substances are likely to end up on the insides of your arteries. But how do levels of blood triglycerides—the total amount of this fat in your blood—help to clarify the picture? Though doctors have been able to measure this blood fat for decades, there is still debate among experts concerning what blood triglycerides can tell us about the likelihood of atherosclerosis. In the last several years this debate has intensified. Medical researchers are hard at work trying to refine our knowledge of how the body processes this fat and to understand the complex relationship between triglycerides and the company they keep in the blood—namely, good and bad cholesterol.

How can we better understand this debate among doctors over the meaning of blood triglycerides? The first step is to take a look at how your body normally uses this fat. We can do this by hitching a ride with triglycerides as they travel through the bloodstream and are broken down by proteins. Triglycerides undergo a fascinating series of changes as they move through the body, making trips through the circulatory system that often begin and end in the liver. These fats are constantly being dismantled and rebuilt as they are metabolized by the body. Triglycerides provide energy for muscles and are used to manufacture a more familiar blood fat, LDL cholesterol. Excess fat molecules are put away in storage for later use in the layers of fat that surround internal organs and line our abdomen or thighs. In Chapter 7 we look at how high triglyceride levels can increase your risk of heart disease.

Q: How do triglycerides get converted into energy?

A: To answer that question, let us take a look at how the triglycerides in our food (the saturated and unsaturated fats discussed in the last chapter) are metabolized after a meal. We will skip ahead to the process of digestion because that is when the story starts to get interesting. During digestion your intestines prepare these fats for their initial entrance into the bloodstream. They do this by creating a number of tiny spherical particles made of triglyceride and cholesterol and coated with protein. You can picture these particles, called chylomicrons, as very tiny balls of fat and cholesterol. If you have ever poured bacon grease or oil into a sink full of water, you have seen this process on a larger scale: The oil forms tiny globules on contact with water. Because your blood consists largely of water, the fat and cholesterol you get from food form tiny balls when released into the bloodstream. The chylomicrons contain much more triglyceride than cholesterol at this stage in the process. When these chylomicrons flood the bloodstream, your blood triglyceride levels begin to climb. This is the reason that doctors require that you fast before a blood test for triglycerides—they do not want this temporary infusion of fat to influence your blood triglyceride measurement or your LDL measurement, which is often calculated using your triglyceride levels instead of being measured directly.

Once in the blood, the tiny balls of fat and cholesterol flow through thousands of miles of blood vessels. It is near the inside linings of vessels, especially in fatty tissue or skeletal muscle, that a two-man team of proteins begins the process of *dismantling* the triglycerides contained in the balls of fat and cholesterol. This protein "duo" is composed of lipoprotein lipase and apo C-II. Together these proteins pluck the fatty acids from the triglycerides. As you recall from Chapter 5, triglycerides are actually "bundles" of smaller fats called fatty acids. These fatty acids, known as the building blocks of fat, are stripped from the triglycerides in order to provide energy for your muscles. Excess fatty acids are transported to fatty tissue for storage. There these fatty acids are put back together again to form triglycerides. Your body reserves the right to dismantle these fats again when necessary in order to provide the body with energy between meals. The breaking down of chylomicrons in the blood takes place very rapidly. These tiny balls of fat and cholesterol are cannibalized by the protein duo within minutes of entering the bloodstream.

◆

Flowchart 1: Chylomicrons

Fat is ingested during a meal.

↓

Your intestines produce tiny spherical particles called chylomicrons by bundling your triglycerides together with cholesterol and protein. These chylomicrons are released into the bloodstream.

↓

In blood vessels, the chylomicrons are "broken down" by a duo of proteins that strips most (but not all) of the fatty acids from these tiny balls of fat and cholesterol. The remaining particles, called very low-density lipoprotein (VLDL) remnants, are smaller in size.

↓

> *The fatty acids freed during this process are used for energy or stored as fat.*

↓

> *Remnants circulate in the blood and eventually are absorbed by the liver.*

◆

Q: So all the triglycerides that I eat are used for energy or put into storage for later use?

A: No, this is only half the story. The journey of triglycerides is not over yet. The protein duo in your bloodstream plucks only a certain amount of fatty acids from the tiny balls of fat and cholesterol. The remaining particles, called remnants, are even smaller in size. When they first enter your blood, the chylomicrons are heavy with triglycerides. After being "mined" of their fatty acids by the two proteins, the remnants contain more *cholesterol* than triglyceride. So what is the next stop for the remnants? They end up in the liver. Here the triglycerides that survived the ravages of the proteins in your bloodstream undergo yet another transformation. The liver uses these triglycerides (as well as some triglyceride it makes on its own) to make VLDL particles, which are sent back into the bloodstream. A VLDL particle exiting the liver contains 80% triglyceride and only 20% cholesterol—this ratio will soon change as VLDL is metabolized. VLDL particles are broken down and reduced in size while in the blood-

stream by the actions of the protein duo. The fatty acids
freed during this process are again used by the body for
energy if needed or put away for storage. Some of the
VLDL broken down in the blood is returned to the
liver. But as you will see later in this chapter, the final
series of steps in the processing of VLDL is important.
After being transformed into some "intermediary" substances and losing much of its triglyceride cargo, some
of the VLDL in your blood is made into LDL cholesterol. As you saw in Chapter 4, most doctors consider
LDL to be the most important blood fat when determining heart disease risk.

◆

Flowchart 2: VLDL Particles

*In the liver, triglycerides are packaged with
cholesterol and protein to form VLDL. These
particles are released into the bloodstream.*

↓

*In blood vessels, VLDL is "broken down" by a
duo of proteins that strips most (but not all)
of the fatty acids from these particles. The
remaining particles, called VLDL remnants,
are smaller in size.*

↓

*The fatty acids freed during this process are used
for energy or stored as fat.*

↓

> *Some of the VLDL remnants circulate in the blood and eventually return to the liver. Others are transformed into intermediate substances and then into LDL cholesterol.*

Remnants: A Role in Plaque Buildup?

The tiny particles known as chylomicrons and the VLDL produced by the liver are known as triglyceride-rich lipoproteins. Before they are broken down in the blood (which occurs rapidly when either of these particles enters the bloodstream), most of their cargo is triglyceride along with a small amount of cholesterol. Referring to them as "triglyceride-rich" helps to distinguish them from the more familiar, cholesterol-carrying particles that we discussed in Chapter 4—namely, HDL cholesterol and LDL cholesterol, which also circulate in the blood. During metabolism, both types of triglyceride-rich lipoproteins are quickly broken down in the bloodstream and most of their fatty acid cargo is mined by the proteins known as lipoprotein lipase and apo C-II. The remaining particles, which contain more cholesterol than triglyceride, are called remnants. They are eventually taken up by the liver. Some of the VLDL remnants undergo a series of changes until they become LDL cholesterol. We need to learn about chylomicron and VLDL remnants in order to understand the role of high triglyceride levels in the development of coronary artery disease (CAD), which is discussed in more detail in the next chapter. These remnant particles may affect your risk of heart disease in direct and indirect ways.

Direct

Like HDL and LDL particles, remnants of chylomicrons and VLDL *do* carry cholesterol. In fact, these remnants actually contain *more* cholesterol than triglyceride. How do remnants contribute to atherosclerosis? Doctors believe that these tiny particles may get trapped in the walls of arteries and unload their cargo of cholesterol. The higher your triglyceride levels, the greater the number of remnants circulating in your blood. Before they are broken down (and reduced in size) in the bloodstream, chylomicrons and VLDL are too large to get trapped in the walls of arteries.

Indirect

The way your body process triglycerides can also affect HDL and LDL cholesterol. It is well known that triglycerides and HDL tend to have an inverse metabolic relationship—when your triglycerides levels are up, your HDL cholesterol tends to be down, and vice versa. Elevated triglycerides may also enhance the plaque-building potential of LDL cholesterol.

• *HDL cholesterol.* It may help to use a simplified metaphor here. For the moment, think of HDL and LDL cholesterol as trains that run in opposite directions. HDL is called good cholesterol because it transports its cargo of cholesterol to the liver (where it is cleared or used to make other substances) and helps to reduce plaque buildup. LDL tends to deposit its larger cargo of fat onto artery walls in a process that we will examine in more detail in Chapter 7. Why do high blood triglycerides go hand in hand with low HDL? Some doctors believe that as remnants and HDL cholesterol circulate in the blood, an excessive amount of cholesterol from HDL is improperly *detoured* into the remnant particles. These remnants may carry the cholesterol back in the *wrong* direction—in other words, onto the walls of arteries.

- *LDL cholesterol.* Doctors also believe that triglycerides may have the power to make a "bad" cholesterol even worse. High triglyceride levels are associated with the production of smaller, denser LDL cholesterol. Why do the size and density of LDL matter? Smaller, denser particles of LDL are more likely to become trapped in the linings of arteries and are thought to be more vulnerable to oxidative changes caused by free radicals. In simple terms, small and dense LDL can lead to greater plaque buildup than "garden variety" LDL.

Doctors are still attempting to understand triglyceride metabolism and its effect on your risk of CAD. The main purpose of this chapter is to give you an overview of how your body processes triglycerides. It also introduces some important terms and concepts and explains how doctors measure your blood levels of this fat. Chapter 7 takes a more in-depth look at how triglycerides may affect your risk of heart disease.

◆

Q: I'm still not sure exactly how triglycerides become body fat. And why is it that I seem to have more fat in some places and not others, no matter how much I exercise?

A: That is a good question. Learning how your body uses triglycerides makes it easier to understand how we gain weight as a result of eating too much and exercising too little. You may even be able to form a mental picture of this process. When you eat too many foods high in fat or calories, you are flooding your bloodstream with triglycerides. How are nonfat calories transformed into fat? Calories not burned by the body are automatically converted into triglycerides, which explains why eating too much of *anything* can lead to weight problems. Excess body fat accumulates when your body is asked to process more triglycerides than it knows what to do with. After using them to create energy and produce other substances needed by the body, what to do with the remaining fat? Ever mindful of the future, your body sends these fats into storage by "stacking them up" in deposits of fatty tissue. It is true that the fatty acids in stored triglycerides can be removed and used to provide energy for your muscles. But if you are not getting enough exercise—exercise *requires* increased energy—most of your body fat will continue to stay right where it is (and where most of us do not want it). Have you ever wondered why you tend to store fat in some places on your body while others do not? Each of us has a genetic predisposition as to *where* we get fat. The reason why body shape varies so much from person to person is that we do not all have the same proportion of fat cells in the same places. Your genetic code determines where on your body to distribute an "overstock" of triglycerides. You may be surprised to learn that the number of fat cells in your body does not actually fluctuate along with changes in weight. The number of fat cells remains fairly constant. The reason we get fatter or thinner is because the fat cells themselves get bigger or smaller.

As most of us are all too aware, these fat cells are not evenly distributed throughout the body. They occur in different amounts in different places. Your elbows, for example, are notoriously free of fat. We are occasionally reminded of this when we strike our "funny bone." Other parts of our bodies, such as the buttocks, abdomen, and thighs, contain larger numbers of fat cells. Some of these variations are related to gender. Men tend to carry extra pounds around the midsection in what are affectionately referred to as love handles. Women tend to experience weight gain in their hips and thighs. Though being over-weight is always a health risk, the so-called "male pattern" of weight distribution is more closely associated with a number of health problems including premature heart disease, diabetes, hypertension, and cancer. There are also differences in fat distribution between members of the same sex. These are genetic differences that we cannot change even by losing weight. Whether we get fatter or thinner, the specific *areas* on our bodies where fat tends to accumulate remains the same. See Chapter 5 for more information on weight gain and obesity.

◆

A Long, Strange Trip: The Journey of Triglycerides Through the Body

Triglycerides are used by the body in different ways and can be "recycled" as needed. The triglycerides that you get from food provide energy for your muscles, are stored as body fat, and are used to make LDL.

- *Down the hatch.* This is the part of the process that we enjoy the most. But it is only after the triglycerides in our food have satisfied our palates that they really get down to work. Once in the intestines, triglycerides are combined with cho-lesterol to produce tiny, protein-coated balls called chylomicrons.
- *Into the bloodstream.* Once the chylomicrons enter the bloodstream, the triglyceride portion is

stripped of its precious cargo of fatty acids. This dismantling of the triglycerides takes place near the inner linings of blood vessels and is carried out by a duo of proteins. Your body burns the fatty acids freed during this process to create energy. Fatty acids not needed by the body for energy are reformed into triglycerides and stored as body fat. The smaller, cannibalized remnants are taken up by the liver.

- *On to the liver.* This is the destination for the remnants. Here the triglycerides that survived the ravages of the proteins in your bloodstream undergo yet another transformation. The liver processes these triglycerides into VLDL.

- *Back into the bloodstream.* VLDL, which is mostly made of triglyceride, is broken down in your blood by the duo of proteins and reduced in size. The remnants of VLDL contain more cholesterol than triglyceride. The fatty acids released during this process are used for energy or stored. Some of the VLDL in your blood undergoes a series of changes until it becomes the more familiar LDL.

◆

Q: How do doctors check triglyceride levels?

A: By means of a blood test. An elastic band or blood pressure cuff will be wrapped snugly around your upper arm in order to cause the veins in your lower arm to swell with blood. A needle is then inserted into a vein on the inside of your arm below your elbow or into one of veins on the back of your hand. Triglycerides can be checked at the same time as your cholesterol levels as long as you have fasted for 12 hours beforehand and had nothing to eat or drink during that time except water. (This test may change in the future, however; see page 122 for the latest information on experimental methods of testing blood triglyceride levels.) You now probably have a better idea of why this fasting is necessary and why it is so important in order to get an accurate reading. As you saw earlier in this chapter, after a meal your triglyceride levels are higher due to the presence of chylomicron remnants in your blood. Blood triglyceride levels continue to rise for several hours after you eat. They peak after four hours and return to normal levels about eight hours after a meal. By that time most of the triglyceride in your blood is in the form of VLDL remnants. Doctors do not measure your blood triglyceride level when your bloodstream is full of chylomicron remnants because this can produce widely varying results depending on what you ate before the test. The "true" measurement—this is the scientific thinking at the moment—reflects the amount of triglycerides circulating in your blood after the chylomicron remnants from recent meals have been cleared. To use an extreme example, imagine for a moment the impact that a burger and fries could have on your triglycerides! At high levels, triglycerides can actually turn blood plasma (a clear, yellowish liquid made mostly of water) a milky white color due to the presence of large amounts of VLDL or chylomicron remnants.

Q: Are there any other factors that can affect the results of my blood triglyceride test?

A: Yes. While you may know the importance of fasting before a blood test for triglycerides, did you know that fluctuations in weight can also affect the measurement? The fact is that the process of losing or gaining weight also influences levels of this blood fat. Triglyceride levels are higher during periods of weight gain and lower when you are losing weight. You should only have your triglyceride levels checked when your weight has been relatively stable for several months before the test. Be sure to always tell your doctor the truth about changes in your weight. Do not be embarrassed to admit that you are trying to lose a few pounds or that you have recently gained some. This sort of vanity only threatens to distort your true blood triglyceride level and may cloud the effort made by you and your doctor to evaluate your risk of heart disease. Pregnancy and certain medications can also alter your test results. Estrogen drugs (including contraceptives) can produce a blood triglyceride measurement that is artificially high. Taking ascorbic acid (vitamin C) or asparaginase (Elspar) may result in a lower triglyceride level.

◆

Are Doctors Measuring Triglyceride Levels the Wrong Way?

Blood triglyceride levels are typically measured in the fasting state. But medical studies of triglyceride levels in the blood after a meal have produced surprising results. These studies suggest that a blood triglyceride measurement taken under controlled conditions after eating (before chylomicron remnants have been cleared from the bloodstream) may actually be a more accurate predictor of the risk of heart disease or the extent of plaque buildup in the coronary arteries. Some doctors even believe that the fasting triglyceride values taken during decades of study may have obscured the meaning of triglycerides as a risk factor for heart disease. Researchers speculate that in the future it may become standard to test for triglycerides after a meal. These measurements may replace those taken in the fasting state or be used to help doctors *refine* their knowledge of how your body is using triglycerides. See Chapter 7 for more information on the significance of postprandial (after-eating) triglyceride measurements.

◆

Triglycerides: The "New" Cholesterol?

*Steve, a high-level executive at a brokerage firm, was
diagnosed with familial combined hyperlipidemia
(FCH) several years ago at the age of 45. This type of
blood fat (also called a blood lipid, which is composed
of cholesterol and triglyceride) disorder was first discovered less than a generation ago by doctors studying
heart attack survivors and their first-degree relatives—
fathers, mothers, siblings, and children. In FCH, members of the same family have different combinations of
elevated blood fats and tend to develop heart disease
early in life (before age 55). Usually the result of inherit-
ing a faulty gene, FCH is associated with increased production of very low-density lipoprotein (VLDL) in the
liver. Steve had a form of FCH in which triglycerides and*

total cholesterol are very high. While he had high levels of VLDL—the precursor of low density lipoprotein (LDL) cholesterol—Steve had a normal amount of LDL (the "bad" cholesterol) because his body was having trouble converting VLDL into LDL. Steve's VLDL was almost 400 mg/dL and his triglycerides were sky high at 1,800 mg/dL. His total cholesterol was almost twice normal at 380 mg/dL. Despite having a desirable level of LDL cholesterol, Steve's total cholesterol measurement was elevated because it included the cholesterol being carried by his excess VLDL, which also carries a certain amount of cholesterol. When your VLDL is very high, the cholesterol it carries can really add up.

After helping Steve to interpret his blood fat levels, he and I crafted a treatment plan designed to lower his triglycerides and improve his overall lipid (fat) profile. This plan included reducing the amount of cholesterol and saturated fat in his diet and starting a program of regular, aerobic exercise. These were big changes for Steve, whose busy work schedule often included lunches with clients several times a week where he was used to choosing foods that were high in saturated fat and cholesterol such as steak, french fries, and dishes made with rich cream sauces. Steve also mentioned that because of his hectic schedule, he often had trouble finding time to exercise. I recommended that Steve limit his intake of saturated fat to less than 7% of his total calories and get no more than 200 mg of cholesterol from the foods he ate. Trimming the fat from his diet helped to slow the production of VLDL in his liver and also made it easier for him to achieve and maintain an ideal weight. Weight reduction was an important part of Steve's treatment program since he was about 25 pounds too heavy. I explained to Steve that safely lowering his weight was important because excess fat is associated with increased output of VLDL. Steve and I also discussed ways in which he might fit exercise into his daily life, such as walking to work instead of taking the bus and getting up a bit earlier in the morning a few days a week to utilize the gym in his office building. Although medications are sometimes prescribed in cases of FCH, Steve and I decided to first see if we could lower his blood fat levels through diet and lifestyle changes.

His commitment to a heart-healthy way of life paid off in less time than he imagined. In just six months Steve lost the extra weight and his lipid profile underwent a major change for the better. His total cholesterol was in the normal range and his triglycerides had dropped a full 1,500 mg/dL. After several years of medication-free treatment, Steve is free of coronary artery disease (CAD) and his blood fat levels are in the desirable range.

Unlike cholesterol, triglycerides are not exactly a hot topic of conversion around the office or in your local diner or coffee shop. They do not grab newspaper headlines or make the TV news. You probably will not find cereals or other food products in your grocery store that claim to reduce your risk of heart disease by helping to lower your triglyceride levels. But all this may soon change. After more than 40 years of study, doctors now believe that triglyceride levels play a more important role in the development of coronary artery disease (CAD) than was previously thought and may help to refine our knowledge of how the body uses cholesterol.

As you saw in Chapter 4, we have long relied on measurements of high-density lipoprotein (HDL) and low-density lipoprotein (LDL) cholesterol to evaluate how our bodies process cholesterol and to predict how much of it will end up where it does not belong—namely, on the insides of arteries. HDL and LDL are the protein "vehicles" that carry cholesterol from one place to another in the body. HDL is referred to as good cholesterol because it removes this waxy substance from the blood and deposits it in the liver, where it is removed from the body or used to make other substances. LDL is known as bad cholesterol because it tends to unload its deposit of cholesterol on artery walls, where it can build up and form plaque. Most efforts to reduce the risk of heart disease focus on lowering LDL cholesterol.

This much you may already know. Most Americans concerned about their risk of heart disease are familiar with HDL and LDL cholesterol and understand how higher or lower levels of these blood fats can affect the buildup of plaque. The goal of this chapter is to explain the importance of those *other* cholesterol-carrying particles in the blood—chylomicrons and very low-density lipoprotein (VLDL). Chylomicrons are the tiny spherical particles made of triglyceride, cholesterol, and protein released into the bloodstream after a meal. VLDL also contains triglyceride, cholesterol, and protein and is produced in the liver. In Chapter 6 we learned two important facts about these particles.

- *Fact 1.* Chylomicrons and VLDL not only transport triglyceride molecules from place to place in the body but also carry a certain amount of cholesterol. After being quickly broken down in the blood and reduced in size, the remnants particles may get trapped in the inner walls of your arteries and unload their cholesterol cargo.
- *Fact 2.* The remnants of chylomicrons and VLDL circulate alongside HDL and LDL in the blood. A certain amount of cholesterol from your HDL—destined for the liver—may be detoured to chylomicron remnants. Because VLDL is used to make

LDL cholesterol, high levels of the former may result in high LDL levels or in tiny, dense forms of LDL. The denser form of bad cholesterol is considered more unhealthy than the garden-variety size.

Doctors measure triglyceride levels—the total amount of this fat in your blood—as well as VLDL in order to better understand how chylomicron and VLDL remnants are affecting the way your body is using cholesterol. In this chapter we are going to put these particles "under the microscope" and take a closer look at how they can deposit cholesterol in your arteries—a fairly recent scientific discovery—or worsen your levels of good and bad cholesterol. We also examine the results of medical studies to better understand the role that elevated triglycerides play in the development of heart disease. Some of this research appears to reveal a cause-and-effect relationship between high triglycerides and CAD while other studies suggest that elevated triglycerides are merely *associated* with cardiovascular disease. While a diet high in fat and cholesterol may boost your blood triglyceride, high triglycerides can also occur when the body fails to process chylomicrons and VLDL remnants properly. These problems with triglyceride metabolism are often inherited but can usually be corrected by diet and lifestyle changes or the use of triglyceride-lowering medication. Chapter 8 for more information on how to reduce your triglyceride levels.

Q: I understand why it's important to lower LDL in the blood. But I'm still not clear what triglycerides have to do with clogged arteries. Can you explain?

A: Yes. But before we explain how elevated triglycerides may affect your risk of heart disease, we should review how arteries become clogged with cholesterol in the first place. Once we understand this process, it is easier to see how chylomicron and VLDL remnants enter the picture.

As you saw Chapter 2, CAD does not suddenly "materialize" at midlife. The process of atherosclerosis, which can lead to CAD later in life, begins during childhood or young adulthood and progresses for decades. The slow-growing plaques that develop during these years are composed mainly of cholesterol. They also contain a number of other substances, including the mineral calcium, fibrin (a substance that helps blood to clot), cellular debris, and more. Over time these hard deposits thicken the wall of an artery, forcing blood to squeeze through a narrower than normal space. Cholesterol is a waxy substance that the body needs for good health. It only presents a problem when large amounts of it accumulate on artery walls. How does it get there? LDL is considered the main culprit. The LDL in your blood tends to get trapped in the inner layer of the arterial wall (called the intima), where it deposits its large cargo of cholesterol. Doctors believe that this process is accelerated when LDL cholesterol becomes oxidized by free radicals, the destructive fragments of oxygen molecules produced as a byproduct when your body's cells use oxygen to burn fat. As cholesterol builds up in the arteries, a special breed of cells (filled with fat and cholesterol) called foam cells are produced. These foam cells make up most of what we call plaque. While LDL deposits cholesterol on artery walls, HDL is busy removing cholesterol from plaque deposits and sending it to the liver, where it is removed from the body or transformed into other substances. HDL may also block the uptake of LDL in the linings of the arteries.

Q: So how do high levels of triglycerides in my blood affect the process of atherosclerosis?
A: In several ways. Elevated triglycerides can worsen your levels of good and bad cholesterol and may also enhance the plaque-building potential of LDL cholesterol. But the big news in triglyceride research is the recent discovery that chylomicron and VLDL remnants in your blood may actually deposit plaque *directly* onto your arteries in the same manner that LDL does.

Good and Bad Cholesterol

Doctors have long known that triglycerides and HDL tend to have an "inverse metabolic relationship." This is a fancy way of saying that when your triglyceride levels are up, your HDL cholesterol tends to be down. Why do high blood triglycerides go hand in hand with low HDL? Some doctors believe that as chylomicron and VLDL remnants circulate in the blood alongside HDL, an excessive amount of cholesterol from HDL is *detoured* into the former particles (at the same time, some of the triglyceride from these particles is transferred to HDL). Doctors also believe that triglycerides may have the power to make a "bad" cholesterol even worse. High triglyceride levels can boost the amount of LDL in the blood and are associated with the production of smaller, denser LDL cholesterol particles. You may be thinking, "But isn't it better to have smaller bad cholesterol?" The answer is *no*. It is better to have *lower numbers* of LDL particles but not *smaller* particles. Extrasmall LDL is considered more potent as a plaque builder because smaller particles of LDL are more likely to become trapped in the linings of arteries. To make matters worse, they are also thought to be more vulnerable to the damage caused by free radicals.

Plaque Buildup

It is important to make a distinction here between full-size chylomicrons and VLDL particles and their *remnants*. The larger versions of these particles—which are broken down into remnants within minutes of entering the bloodstream—are not thought to play a direct role in the development of atherosclerosis. In other words, your blood levels of these cholesterol-carrying particles may affect your good and bad cholesterol measurements but they do not unload their cholesterol directly onto your artery walls. Remnants are a different story. Recent research suggests that chylomicron and VLDL remnants do get trapped in the walls of arteries and unload their cargo of cholesterol. Cholesterol that reaches the intima by way of these remnants may be used to make new foam cells—and that results in more artery-clogging plaque. These remnants may be vulnerable to oxidation, in which case they pose an even greater threat. *This bears repeating: Chylomicron and VLDL remnants may be able to deposit cholesterol onto your artery walls in the same manner that LDL does.* When your triglyceride levels are high, there are larger number of these remnants in your blood and a greater risk that your arteries are being exposed to their LDL-like effects. The length of time these particles spend in your bloodstream (before being sent to the liver) can also affect the risk of plaque buildup—the longer they circulate, the greater the risk. Studies suggest that the LDL-like effects of chylomicron and VLDL remnants may have the most impact during the early stages of plaque formation.

◆
Your Triglyceride Vocabulary

HDL and LDL cholesterol are familiar terms to
most people concerned about their risk of developing clogged arteries. Here are some new words to
add to your "heart vocabulary."

- *Blood triglycerides*—this is a measurement of the
  total amount of triglyceride in your blood. It is
  taken in the fasting state. Doctors can measure
  levels of VLDL in your blood as well.
- *Chylomicrons*—these tiny spherical particles
  composed of triglyceride, cholesterol, and protein
  are released into the bloodstream in large numbers after a meal. Once in the bloodstream, chylomicrons are broken down into remnant particles
  within minutes. Most of those particles are usually cleared by the liver after 10 to 12 hours.
- *VLDL*—these particles—which contain five
  times as much triglyceride as cholesterol—are
  made in the liver. After being broken down in the
  blood, some of the remnant particles are transformed into intermediary substances that become
  LDL cholesterol. LDL is considered the main
  culprit in plaque buildup.
- *Remnants*—this is the term used to describe what
  remains of chylomicrons and VLDL after they
  are broken down and reduced in size by a duo of
  proteins in the blood. Many doctors now believe
  that these cholesterol-carrying remnants get
  trapped in the inner linings of arteries, where they
  deposit their cargo of cholesterol. Like LDL cholesterol, remnants of chylomicrons and VLDL
  may be damaged by free radicals. This makes
  them more potent as plaque builders.

- *Lipoprotein lipase and apo C-II*—this protein duo is responsible for breaking down chylomicrons and VLDL. The duo strips these particles of their fatty acids as they pass through blood vessels in fatty tissue, skeletal muscle, the pericardium (the thin, protective membrane that surrounds the heart), and breast tissue in women.

◆

Q: I've heard that triglycerides are a matter of controversy in the medical community. Some doctors think that they are an important risk factor for heart disease while others don't. What's the story?

A: This is a very good question with a not so simple answer. It is true that triglycerides are still something of a controversy among doctors and that our knowledge of this blood fat is still evolving. All doctors agree that lowering triglycerides is necessary in certain situations—for example, if your levels are sky-high or if you have one of the inherited disorders described later in this chapter that prevent your body from processing blood fats in a normal fashion. But there is less agreement about the importance of the borderline-high triglyceride levels that doctors see on a fairly regular basis and whether elevated triglycerides increase the likelihood of heart disease in the absence of other risk factors. Some experts claim that medical studies have failed to establish a cause-and-effect relationship between high triglycerides and cardiovascular disease. They believe that elevated triglycerides are merely *associated* with CAD or are important mainly as an *indicator* that your body has trouble processing more familiar blood fats such as HDL and LDL. But as you have seen earlier in this chapter, new research suggests that chylomicron and VLDL remnants in your blood can

actually cause plaque buildup *directly* by depositing cholesterol on artery walls. If the latter view becomes well
accepted, an elevated triglyceride level may be recognized as an important risk factor for heart disease even in
the absence of other factors—what doctors refer to as an
independent risk factor.

Why do some medical studies suggest that elevated
triglycerides are an important risk factor for CAD while
others do not? This is a complicated question that is still
being debated among experts. The issue is made more
complex by the fact that people with elevated levels of
this blood fat often have a number of other risk factors for
heart disease. These include low HDL, high LDL, and
existing medical conditions such as hypertension and diabetes. Sorting out these other factors and isolating the
significance of triglycerides has led to mixed results.
While we cannot go into much detail here due to the technical nature of the debate, we can point out two factors
that may be obscuring our view of how important triglycerides really are. Both factors relate to the way doctors
measure blood triglycerides.

Fasting or After Meals?

Medical studies that take triglyceride levels into
account have always relied on fasting values of this blood
fat. But new studies in the last decade or so are question-
ing the wisdom of this approach. Research suggests that
postprandial (after-eating) triglyceride levels—taken
before most of the chylomicron remnants have been
cleared from the bloodstream—may be better able to predict the risk of CAD or the extent of plaque buildup than
levels taken after a 12-hour fast. In these studies, high
postprandial triglyceride levels appear to be a strong and

independent risk factor for heart disease. Some doctors even believe that the fasting triglyceride values taken during decades of study may have obscured the significance of high triglycerides as a CAD risk factor. Researchers speculate that in the future it may become standard to test for triglycerides after a meal. These measurements may replace those taken in the fasting state or be used to help doctors *refine* their knowledge of how your body is processing triglycerides.

The Devil Is in the Details

The way we measure blood triglycerides fails to take several important variables into account. They include the size of chylomicron and VLDL remnants, their number, and the amount of cholesterol that they carry. Why do these variables matter? The smaller the remnant particles are, the more likely it is that they will get trapped in artery walls. Remember—when it comes to remnants (and LDL cholesterol), smaller is *not* better. Taking a "headcount" of these remnants in order to find out how many there are in the blood would also be helpful in assessing risk. Finally, doctors would like to know how much cholesterol is being carried by chylomicron and VLDL remnants. If their cholesterol content is higher than normal, they may be depositing larger amounts of cholesterol on vessel walls. As you can see, any of these variables may obscure the true significance of a blood triglyceride level. We can illustrate this point with a simple example. Suppose you and a friend have the same blood triglyceride level. This suggests that you both have the same degree of heart disease risk, speaking *strictly* in terms of triglycerides and not taking account of other risk factors. But this assumption could actually be false.

One of you may be at greater risk due to a larger number of remnant particles that carry more cholesterol than usual.

◆

Triglyceride-Level Guidelines

If your doctor has not checked your triglycerides along with your cholesterol levels, ask why. It is especially important to have your triglycerides measured if you have CAD, a family history of premature heart disease (before age 55), high total cholesterol (200 mg/dL or higher), desirable total cholesterol (less than 200 mg/dL) accompanied by two CAD risk factors, or a medical condition such as diabetes or pancreatitis (inflammation of the pancreas).

- Normal triglycerides: Less than 200 mg/dL.
- Borderline-high triglycerides: 200 to 400 mg/dL.
- High triglycerides: 400 to 1,000 mg/dL.
- Very high triglycerides: Greater than 1,000 mg/dL.

Source: The Second Expert Panel on the Detection, Evaluation, and Treatment of High Blood Cholesterol in Adults (Adult Treatment Panel II). National Cholesterol Education Program, National Institutes of Health, National Heart, Lung, and Blood Institute, NIH Publication No. 93-3095, September 1993.

◆

Q: As a layperson, how can I have a meaningful discussion with my doctor about my triglyceride level?
A: That is a great question. The fact is you do not need a medical degree in order to talk to your doctor about the

meaning of your blood triglyceride level. You have already taken a more active role in your own health care by reading this book and becoming more informed about this blood fat. The next step is to bridge the "communication gap" that often exists between doctor and patient. Here are a few questions you can ask your doctor in order to get the ball rolling.

- What are your views about blood triglycerides and the risk of heart disease?
- Do you believe it is important to check my triglyceride level? If not, why not?
- Do you believe that triglycerides are an independent risk factor for CAD?
- Do you keep up with the current research regarding triglycerides?
- What is the significance of medical studies that suggest high triglycerides can increase the risk of heart disease?
- What does my blood triglyceride level really mean?
- What measures can I take to reduce my triglyceride level?

Do not hesitate to take the initiative and ask your doctor questions about your care. A good doctor has the ability and willingness to explain medical concepts in simple, understandable terms and will not mind taking the time to help you interpret your triglyceride levels. Bringing a list of questions or discussion points to the doctor's office shows that you take your health seriously. You can use some of the information in this chapter when talking to your doctor. If your doctor has pamphlets or other helpful literature, take this material home with you and read it thoroughly. Talking to doctors with different points of view is another great way to stay informed.

Q: Do high triglyceride levels have any special significance for older women?

A: Many doctors believe that high triglycerides are an important risk factor in postmenopausal women. This view is supported by several medical studies. One of these is the well-known Framingham Heart Study, an ongoing research project involving more than 5,000 men and women from the small town of Framingham, Massachusetts. The Framingham Study has played a key role in identifying most of the heart-disease risk factors that we discussed in Chapter 3, such as high cholesterol, hypertension, smoking, diabetes, and obesity. So what does this study tell us about triglyceride levels in older women? At a 14-year follow-up, researchers found a strong connection between high triglyceride levels and CAD in women between the ages of 50 and 69 (most women experience menopause around age 50). The findings suggest that elevated triglycerides may be a significant and independent risk factor in this group, even when other factors, such as hypertension and smoking, are accounted for. Women who had high triglycerides paired with low HDL cholesterol were *twice* as likely to develop CAD as those who did not have this blood fat combination. High triglycerides were also found to be an important risk factor in a recent meta-analysis (an analysis of a number of previous medical studies) involving more than 10,000 older women studied for an average of 11 years. When "isolated" as a risk factor, elevated triglycerides appeared to increase the risk of heart disease in these women by almost 40%. Some doctors speculate that estrogen's ability to reduce the risk of heart disease in postmenopausal women may be partly due to the fact that it can speed the clearance of chylomicron and VLDL remnants from the blood (even though estrogen also increases the production of VLDL). This may reduce the time that arteries are exposed to these cholesterol-carrying particles.

Q: How do high triglyceride levels impact older men?

A: Middle-aged and older men with elevated triglycerides are at increased risk for CAD according to a number of medical studies. In some of these studies, high triglycerides appear to be a bigger risk factor for heart disease than high total cholesterol.

- The Copenhagen Male Study involved almost 3,000 initially healthy men between the ages of 53 and 74 who were followed for eight years. After accounting for a number of other risk factors, including HDL and LDL cholesterol, researchers found that men in the study who had the highest triglyceride levels were almost *twice* as likely to develop heart disease as those with normal levels of the blood fat. High triglycerides were found to be an independent risk factor in this study.

- In a meta-analysis involving over 45,000 men who were followed for about eight years, elevated triglycerides appeared to increase the risk of heart disease in these men by almost 15% once the blood fat was "isolated" as a risk factor.

- Over a 14-year period, men participating in the Framingham Heart Study who had high triglycerides and low HDL cholesterol were almost *twice* as likely to develop CAD as men who did not have this blood fat combination.

- Conducted in the United Kingdom, the Collaborative Heart Disease Studies project involved

5,000 men between the ages of 45 and 63 who were in good health when the study began. After about four years, 250 of these men were diagnosed with cardiovascular disease. Researchers found that men with the highest triglyceride levels were about *twice* as likely to develop heart disease as those with the lowest levels of this blood fat, even when other factors such as HDL and total cholesterol were taken into account. In this study, elevated triglycerides outweigh high cholesterol as a risk factor for heart disease.

Q: What is familial combined hyperlipidemia and what does it have to do with triglycerides?
A: The 500,000 Americans with familial combined hyperlipidemia (FCH) have a problem processing triglycerides. The result can be high levels of triglyceride or cholesterol. This inherited blood fat disorder was first discovered less than a generation ago by doctors studying heart attack survivors and their first-degree relatives—fathers, mothers, siblings, and children. These researchers found that, in some cases, members of the same family had different *combinations* of elevated blood fats. For example, a father may have had high triglyceride and total cholesterol levels while his son had elevated LDL and total cholesterol. People with FCH have high levels of triglyceride or cholesterol (or both) because their livers are making too much VLDL. This VLDL overload occurs due to a faulty gene that is passed from parent to child. FCH is associated with premature heart disease and with blood fat levels that fluctuate without explanation. If you are diagnosed with FCH, it is likely that half of your first-degree relatives suffer from the disorder as well—about 33% of this group will probably have high cholesterol, 33% will have high triglyc-

erides, and the rest will have a combination of the two. Why is it that this one disorder results in *different* blood fat problems? The answer has to do with the way that the body processes the excess of VLDL. The rate and mechanism by which VLDL is metabolized (as well as the composition of VLDL as it leaves the liver) determines which fats are elevated.

Slow Processing of VLDL

This results in high triglyceride and total cholesterol levels accompanied by normal LDL cholesterol. Triglycerides are elevated due to the large number of VLDL particles in the blood. The total cholesterol measurement is high because it includes the cholesterol being carried by the excess VLDL. As you have seen earlier in this chapter, VLDL carries a certain amount of cholesterol in addition to its triglyceride cargo. When your VLDL is very high, the cholesterol it bears can really add up. You may be thinking, "If levels of VLDL are elevated, that means LDL cholesterol should be high as well." Your instincts are correct, but in this case the answer is no. Despite the excess of VLDL, people with FCH who have this blood fat profile actually have normal levels of LDL cholesterol because their bodies are not converting VLDL into LDL fast enough.

Normal Processing of VLDL

So what happens if you have FCH and your body transforms the excess VLDL into LDL at a *normal* rate? This scenario really "lights up" your blood fat profile across the board, resulting in high levels of triglycerides, LDL cholesterol, and total cholesterol. Why?

Triglycerides are elevated due to the large number of VLDL particles in the blood. LDL cholesterol is high because large numbers of VLDL particles are being converted into LDL. The total cholesterol measurement mainly reflects the large amount of cholesterol being carried by LDL.

Speedy Processing of VLDL

Some people with FCH have *normal* triglyceride levels, but their total cholesterol and LDL cholesterol are high. This profile is the result when the body breaks down the excess VLDL faster than usual. The combination of too much VLDL and extra-fast conversion of VLDL into LDL results in a high LDL level. Despite the excess VLDL, triglycerides are in the normal range due to the fact that they are metabolized quickly and removed from the blood. Total cholesterol is high in people with this profile because of the large amount of cholesterol being carried by LDL.

How can you tell if you have FCH? Fluctuating blood fat levels are one distinguishing feature of this disorder. A person with FCH may experience (for no apparent reason) a rise or fall in different blood fats over a period of several months. You and your doctor should also investigate the possibility of FCH if you were diagnosed with heart disease at a young age or if you have a family history of premature heart disease. If FCH is suspected, other members of your family (including children) should have their cholesterol and triglyceride levels checked even if they appear to be in good health. The youngest members of your family may need to have their blood fat levels monitored closely as they get older in order to spot trouble early.

Treatment of FCH focuses on slowing the production of VLDL in the liver, since this is the root cause of the high triglyceride or cholesterol levels. This can be accomplished in several ways. If you have FCH, your doctor will recommend that you limit the amount of cholesterol, total fat, and saturated fat in your diet. A high-fat diet only encourages the liver to produce more VLDL. Reducing fat intake helps to slow the production of VLDL and makes it easier to achieve and maintain an ideal weight. Weight reduction is an important part of treatment in people who are obese or have less severe weight problems because excess fat is also associated with increased output of VLDL by the liver. When medication is required to improve the lipid (blood fat) profile of someone with FCH, nicotinic acid (niacin) or a fibric acid derivative is often prescribed because each of these drugs slows the production of VLDL. Because most people with FCH have elevations of different blood fats, more than one lipid-lowering medication may be used to improve your profile. These drug combinations are usually composed of a statin medication paired with either nicotinic acid or the fibric acid derivative gemfibrozil (Lopid).

Q: What is familial hypertriglyceridemia?
A: People with this inherited disorder have high triglyceride and VLDL levels but normal levels of LDL cholesterol. Familial hypertriglyceridemia (FHT) is also associated with a low HDL level that results in an unhealthy ratio of LDL to HDL. This type of blood fat pattern can occur in FCH as well but there are several telltale distinctions between the two disorders. If you have FHT, several of your blood relatives will also have the *same* blood fat pattern. By comparison, family mem-

bers with FCH usually have *different combinations* of elevated blood fats. The lipid profile associated with FHT is also more stable—it does not fluctuate significantly over short periods of time without explanation. In FHT, the liver produces a normal number of VLDL particles but they are abnormally large. These extra-large VLDL particles are "overloaded" with triglyceride molecules. Because the number of VLDL particles made by the liver is normal—only their size is abnormal—the amount of LDL cholesterol is usually normal as well. Though people with FHT often have desirable levels of LDL cholesterol, LDL may become elevated if other risk factors are present. Obesity, for example, can increase the liver's output of these extra-large VLDL particles and boost the amount of LDL cholesterol in the blood. In FHT, triglyceride levels usually become elevated during adolescence or young adulthood and range between 200 and 500 mg/dL. Heavy drinking, estrogen medications, poorly managed diabetes, or hypothyroidism can boost triglyceride levels to 1,000 mg/dL or higher in people with FHT. Beside its effect on triglyceride levels, FHT also increases the risk of developing diabetes or gout. A strict dietary regimen is not only effective in improving blood fat levels in people with FHT but may also reduce the risk of developing diabetes. In you already have diabetes, the diet and lifestyle modifications aimed at lowering your triglyceride levels may help you to better manage your condition and reduce your dependence on insulin medication. Nicotinic acid and gemfibrozil (or other fibric acid derivatives) may be used to help lower triglyceride levels in people with FHT.

◆

Type 3 Hyperlipoproteinemia

People with this rare, inherited disorder usually have high triglyceride and total cholesterol levels. Type 3 hyperlipoproteinemia is associated with obesity and hypothyroidism and often results in premature CAD or peripheral vascular (blood vessel) disease. The disorder is passed from parent to child via a mutated gene. This gene affects the structure of a protein called apo E that is present in the remnants of chylomicrons and VLDL. Because the apo E carried by these remnants is flawed in people with type 3 hyperlipoproteinemia, the liver does not "recognize" the remnants. As a result, the liver does not adequately absorb chylomicron and VLDL remnants and they build up in the blood. The VLDL particles made by the liver may also be "overloaded" with cholesterol. As you saw in Chapter 6, VLDL normally carries about five times as much triglyceride as cholesterol. But in people with this disorder, VLDL may contain *equal* amounts of triglyceride and cholesterol. It is the cholesterol carried by large numbers of chylomicron and VLDL remnants—as opposed to the fat transported by LDL—that causes total cholesterol to be so high in people with this disorder. How high? In people with type 3 hyperlipoproteinemia, deposits of cholesterol and triglyceride may be visible just under the skin. These deposits appear as reddish-yellow streaks or bumps (called xanthomas) on the hands, elbows, or knees. About 80% of people with type 3 hyperlipoproteinemia have xanthomas. Treatment of this disorder includes a low-fat, low-cholesterol diet and weight reduction if necessary. A medication such as gemfibrozil, clofibrate (Atromid-S), or fenofibrate (Tricor) is often needed in order to reduce production of VLDL and increase the effectiveness of the protein duo, which subsequently helps the body break down the excess triglycerides faster so they do not build up in your blood. Treatment is usually successful at reducing the risk of heart disease.

◆

Q: At his last doctor visit, my husband was told that he had an inherited disease called type 5 hyperlipoproteinemia—his triglyceride level was 3,200 mg/dL. Can you tell me more about this disease? Are our children at risk for it as well?

A: People with type 5 hyperlipoproteinemia, which strikes about 1 in 10,000 Americans, have large numbers of chylomicrons and VLDL in their blood because their bodies are not processing them and clearing them from the bloodstream at a normal rate. The problem? The body produces an excess of VLDL and chylomicron particles, and those particles are not broken down fast enough by the body. Some experts speculate that lipotrotein lipase or apo C-II—the proteins that break down triglycerides in the blood—are not present in proper amounts or are not working properly in people with type 5 hyperlipoproteinemia. In some people with diabetes any factor (obesity, for example) that increases the *number* of VLDL particles being produced by the liver worsens the condition. After all, the duo of proteins is not able to sufficiently break down a normal amount of VLDL, let alone an excess of the particles. People with this disorder often have desirable levels of LDL because their VLDL is not being converted into bad cholesterol at the usual speed. But even when their LDL cholesterol levels are normal, people with type 5 hyperlipoproteinemia are at increased risk for atherosclerosis because their arteries are being exposed to large numbers of chylomicron and VLDL remnants. As you have seen earlier in this chapter, these particles may unload their cargo of cholesterol on artery walls and increase the risk of CAD. Unfortunately, there is a strong chance that your children will develop this same type of disorder or a less severe problem with triglyceride metabolism. The good news is that treatment can often bring the high triglyceride levels associated with this disorder under control. Weight reduction is usually the primary goal since people with type 5 hyperlipoproteinemia tend to be overweight or obese. A low-fat diet and lifestyle changes paired with a medication such as clofibrate can bring triglycerides into the normal range in a matter of just a few months.

How to Lower Your Triglyceride Levels

*Jason, age 52, is a corporate lawyer who first came to
see me a year ago. Jason was about 15 pounds overweight at the time and tended to eat his meals on the run
due to his busy schedule. Jason's lipid (blood fat) profile
showed that his low-density lipoprotein (LDL) cholesterol level was normal at 120 mg/dL. His total cholesterol level was also in the desirable range, but his
triglycerides and high-density lipoprotein (HDL) cholesterol levels were in need of some improvement. His
triglycerides were borderline-high at 280 mg/dL and his
HDL (good) cholesterol was borderline low. Jason's
blood pressure was normal and he was in good general
health. When I asked him if he exercised, Jason
explained that his responsibilities at work and at home
left him little time for physical activity except for an*

occasional work-related game of golf. Jason did not consider himself overweight and was surprised when I explained that even an excess of 15 pounds could increase his risk of heart disease. I told Jason that by reducing the fat and cholesterol in his diet and making exercise a regular part of his routine, we could probably lower his triglycerides and raise his HDL cholesterol in a matter of months and reduce his risk of developing coronary artery disease (CAD). Jason agreed to give it a try. He cut back on foods high in cholesterol and limited his intake of dietary fat to 30% of calories. Jason had been a college athlete during his law school days, so the transition from a sedentary to a more active way of life was easy for him once he made exercise a priority. He started jogging three times a week and also lifted weights. He and his wife even began taking brisk walks after dinner. Within six months Jason was at his ideal weight and his triglyceride level had fallen by 85 mg/dL to a healthy 195mg/dL. His HDL cholesterol had also risen to healthy levels. Instead of doing business on the golf course, Jason now suggests a game of racquetball to his clients. After one year, Jason's entire lipid profile had improved and he was feeling better than ever about his health as well as his new leaner look.

This chapter is your guide to preventing or lowering elevated triglycerides. Because triglycerides are the main way that nature "packages" fat, blood levels of triglyceride can often be reduced by limiting the amount of fat that you get from food. By gradually making changes in your diet and getting more exercise, you may be able to lower your levels of this blood fat and reduce your risk of developing coronary artery disease (CAD). Your triglyceride-lowering plan should include cutting back on cholesterol and saturated fat, maintaining a desirable weight, and eliminating unhealthy habits like smoking and drinking alcohol. Most of us know from experience that bad health habits tend to go hand in hand. What may not be so obvious is that healthy behavior can also reinforce itself. For example, eating right and exercising lead to weight loss. Being at or near your ideal weight, in turn, makes exercising easier. Exercise can help reduce your reliance on drugs such as nicotine and alcohol—and so on.

What if diet and exercise fail to lower your triglycerides? If this is the case, your doctor has a variety of medications that can help. Medications may also be considered at the start if your triglyceride levels are high enough—500 mg/dL is generally considered the threshold—or if you already have CAD. Drugs used to improve your lipid (blood fat) profile are referred to as lipid-lowering medications. They are also called "cholesterol-lowering" drugs despite the fact that many of them can be used to lower triglyceride levels as well as the more familiar cholesterol-carrying particles such as high-density lipoprotein (HDL) cholesterol and low-density lipoprotein (LDL) cholesterol. If you have a combination of elevated blood fats—for example, perhaps your LDL cholesterol is high as well as your triglycerides—your doctor may recommend more than one drug in order to improve your lipid profile as a whole.

Q: What is the first step in lowering my triglycerides?
A: Adopting a low-fat, low-cholesterol diet and avoiding simple sugars are great ways to start. You can reduce your triglycerides (as well as your cholesterol levels) and lower your risk of heart disease by eating a diet rich in fruits and vegetables, avoiding meat or eating lean cuts

of it, cutting back on high-fat junk food, avoiding simple sugars such as cane sugar and those found in honey and fruit juices, and reading labels in order to avoid foods high in cholesterol and saturated fat. As you have seen earlier in this book, cholesterol is the main ingredient of artery-clogging plaque. It is found only in foods that come from animals—meats, poultry, fish and other seafood, and dairy products. Egg yolks, organ meats, and shrimp contain especially high amounts. On the other hand, fruits, vegetables, grains, nuts, and other plant foods are naturally cholesterol-free. Saturated fat is so named because it contains a large proportion of hydrogen-rich, saturated fatty acids. Along with the cholesterol that you get from food, saturated fat can raise your blood cholesterol levels more than anything else in your diet. Like cholesterol, saturated fat is found in meat and dairy products. Beef, pork, veal, poultry, butter, milk, and cheese all contain saturated fat as well as cholesterol. Certain oils derived from plants also contain high amounts of saturated fat. These include coconut oil, palm kernel oil, and palm oil (known collectively as tropical oils). Tropical oils are frequently used in the making of potato chips and other processed snack foods.

◆

How to Stick to Your Low-Fat Diet When Eating Out

Having trouble eating right when dining out, these tips may help.

- Choose restaurants that have low–saturated fat, low-cholesterol menu choices. Do not hesitate to make special requests—it is your right as a paying customer.

- Control serving sizes by asking for a side-dish or appetizer-size serving, sharing a dish with a companion, or taking a portion home with you.
- Ask that gravy, butter, rich sauces, and salad dressing be served on the side. That way, you can control the amount of saturated fat and cholesterol that you eat.
- Ask to substitute a salad or baked potato for chips, fries, coleslaw, or other extras—or just ask that the extras be left off of your plate.
- When ordering pizza, order vegetable toppings like green pepper, onions, and mushrooms instead of meat or extra cheese. To make your pizza even lower in fat, order it with half of the cheese or no cheese.
- At fast-food restaurants, choose some of the healthier options such as salads or grilled (not fried or breaded) skinless chicken sandwiches. Go easy on the regular salad dressings and fatty sauces. Limit jumbo or deluxe burgers or sandwiches and avoid french fries.

Source: Adapted from the National Cholesterol Education Program (NCEP): http://rover.nhlbi.nih.gov/chd/Tipsheets/diningout.htm

◆

Q: But how does eating a low-fat diet actually reduce my triglyceride levels?

A: Remember: The fat and cholesterol in your diet are ultimately transformed into chylomicron and very low-density lipoprotein (VLDL) remnants in your blood—the particles that carry triglyceride and cholesterol. When you eat meals high in fat, your bloodstream can become flooded with chylomicron remnants. These particles may unload their cargo of cholesterol onto artery walls. Cholesterol and dietary fats are also used by your liver to make VLDL. As you saw in Chapter 7, VLDL particles eventually become LDL cholesterol after being broken down by proteins in your blood. Like the remnants of chylomicrons, VLDL remnants may also deposit cholesterol in your arteries. In high amounts, VLDL may also increase your LDL levels and result in the formation of dense LDL cholesterol—an extra-potent form of bad cholesterol that increases your risk of atherosclerosis (narrowing and hardening of the arteries) even more than the garden-variety LDL particles. To help lower your triglyceride levels, limit your average daily intake of dietary cholesterol to 300 mg a day—if you already have CAD you should consume no more than 200 mg. You should also limit your intake of saturated fat to 10% of your total calories, in some cases your doctor may recommend that you consume even less. Chapters 6 and 7 for more information about how the body processes triglycerides and why high levels of this blood fat may contribute to the development of CAD.

◆

Trimming the Fat: The Step I and Step II Diets

If you are diagnosed with elevated triglycerides, your doctor may recommend a Step I or Step II diet. These dietary regimens are endorsed by the American Heart Association (AHA) and the National Cholesterol Education Program (NCEP). They can help to lower your blood levels of triglyceride, LDL cholesterol, and total cholesterol while promoting good nutrition.

Recommended Intake as Percent of Total Calories

Nutrient*	Step I Diet	Step II Diet
Total fat	30% or less	30% or less
Saturated fat	8–10%	7% or less
Polyunsaturated fat	Up to 10%	Up to 10%
Monounsaturated fat	Up to 15%	Up to 15%
Carbohydrate	55% or more	55% or more
Protein	Approximately 15%	Approximately 15%
Cholesterol	Less than 300 mg a day	Less than 200 mg a day
Total Calories	To achieve and maintain desired weight	To achieve and maintain desired weight

*Calories from alcohol not included.

What Are Recommended Amounts of Total Fat and Saturated Fat in Grams?

Calorie Level	Total Fat (g)	Step I Diet Saturated Fat (g)	Step II Diet Saturated Fat (g)
1,200	40 or less	11–13	less than 9
1,500	50 or less	13–17	less than 12
1,800	60 or less	16–20	less than 14

Calorie Level	Total Fat (g)	Step I Diet Saturated Fat (g)	Step II Diet Saturated Fat (g)
2,000	67 or less	18–22	less than 16
2,200	73 or less	20–24	less than 17
2,500	83 or less	22–28	less than 19
3,000	100 or less	27-33	less than 23

Source: Reproduced with permission. Heart and Stroke A-Z Guide, 1999. http://www.amhrt.org/Heart_and_Stroke_A_Z_Guide/step1.html. Copyright American Heart Association.

◆

Q: Is it true that alcohol can raise my triglycerides?
A: Yes, this is true. You are probably thinking, "But doesn't alcohol help to *prevent* heart disease?" As you saw Chapter 4, studies do suggest that people who drink moderately—one or two drinks a day for men and one drink daily for women—have lower rates of heart disease than nondrinkers. The one or two drinks of liquor a day (one drink is 12 ounces of beer or 4 ounces of wine) appear to offer a protective effect by possibly boosting HDL cholesterol levels. The problem is that drinking can also increase your triglyceride levels at the same time. The effect of alcohol on your triglycerides may not be a problem if your levels of this blood fat are in the normal range. But if you have elevated levels, your doctor will probably recommend that you eliminate alcohol from your diet altogether— at least until your triglycerides have fallen. As you have seen earlier in this book, there are better ways to

help prevent heart disease than drinking alcohol. The fact is that most doctors and national health organizations do not recommend drinking alcohol to prevent heart disease due to the many health problems associated with drinking. Besides raising triglycerides, alcohol can contribute to hypertension (high blood pressure) and obesity. It can also increase your risk of alcoholism, osteoporosis, and stroke. The bottom line? If you have elevated triglycerides, you can help to lower your levels by reducing the amount of alcohol you drink or by eliminating liquor from your diet altogether. Ask your doctor to help you weigh the potential benefits and risks of moderate drinking. You and your doctor should take your triglyceride level into account as well as your risk for diseases that are associated with alcohol use.

Q: I have diabetes. Do you have any special advice for me?
A: People with diabetes mellitus either have difficulty producing insulin or develop a resistance to the hormone, depending on which form of the disease they have. Insulin helps to convert glucose (blood sugar) into energy and also regulates the way your body absorbs and stores other nutrients and fat that you get from food. People with diabetes are much more likely to have high triglycerides and low HDL cholesterol. In fact, people with type 2 diabetes are *twice* as likely to have elevated triglyceride levels than those without the disease. While there is no cure for diabetes, properly managing your condition not only helps to avoid serious complications but can also reduce your triglyceride level. You can accomplish this by a strict adherence to the low-fat dietary regimen that you and your doctor or registered dietician crafted

together. This diet usually avoids simple sugars such as cane sugar and those found in honey and fruit juices. Exercise is also an important part of controlling your glucose levels. It is especially important for people with diabetes to talk to their doctors before starting a regular program of exercise (see Exercise Tips for People with Diabetes, below) and to wear a medical ID bracelet while working out. Diabetes is associated with vision problems, kidney disorders, and heart disease, and any of these health problems may put practical limits on your exercise routine. You should also monitor your glucose levels before and after exercise in order to evaluate how your body is responding to physical stress. Managing diabetes also means taking your medication (if any), maintaining an ideal weight, avoid smoking and exposure to secondhand smoke, and controlling high blood pressure.

◆

Exercise Tips for People with Diabetes

- Wear proper shoes and check feet before and after exercise.
- Avoid exercising in extremely hot or cold weather. Instead, do your workout in a climate-controlled environment such as your home or a gym. You should also avoid exercise during periods of poor glycemic control.
- People with active proliferative retinopathy should avoid weight lifting, high-impact aerobic activities, and head-down positions.
- People with peripheral neuropathy or circulatory problems should avoid weight-bearing exercises such as running. Try cycling, swimming, or walking instead.

- People with hypertension should avoid weight lifting or other activities that involve straining, such as isometric exercises.

Source: Exercise tips are adapted from Cefalu W. T.: *Practical Guide to Diabetes Management.* Medical Information Press, New York, 1998.

◆

Q: Why is exercise important for lowering my triglycerides?

A: Exercise is important for a number of reasons. As you saw in the introduction to this chapter, many of the steps that you can take to improve your blood-fat levels reinforce each other. Aerobic exercise, which conditions the heart and lungs by making the body work harder to meet the increased oxygen demands of the body, is a key part of your effort to burn fat and calories and maintain a desirable weight. By exercising regularly, you can lower your triglycerides and help raise your levels of HDL cholesterol by up to 20%. Exercise can also be helpful in reducing your dependence on alcohol or cigarettes. The fact is that most of us already know exercise is good for us, but we find excuses to avoid it. The good news is that exercise does not have be a chore or even a solitary activity. Exercise is a great way to spend time with your children and spouse. Try roller skating or mountain biking with your kids. Take brisk walks with your spouse after breakfast and dinner or rekindle your romantic spirit with dancing. Most of my patients start an exercise program for health reasons but continue to stick with it because they see results in their daily lives. They report that they have more energy and less stress. They appreciate the way exercise improves their mood and helps them stay slim without resorting to "starvation" diets. Exercise can help to prevent atherosclerosis and obesity or other weight problems, it can boost blood levels of HDL cholesterol while lowering triglycerides, and can aid in the management of hypertension and diabetes. For all these reasons, physical activity should be a routine part of our lives from childhood to our most advanced years. To lower triglycerides and protect the cardiovascular system from disease, you should get about 30 minutes of aerobic exercise on most days of the week. At least three days a week of heart-pumping exercise are needed to provide significant cardiovascular benefit. Always talk to your doctor about the exercise program you plan to start, especially if you have CAD, diabetes, or other existing medical conditions. Your doctor can explain how to get the most out of your workout and how to exercise safely. See Chapter 3 for more information on exercise, including a list of aerobic activities.

◆

Diet and Lifestyle Changes That Help to Lower Triglycerides

- Trim the fat from your diet (see page 86).
- Maintain the "ideal" weight for your body type and height (see page 95).
- Exercise aerobically at least 30 minutes a day, most days of the week (see page 54).
- Stop drinking alcohol (see page 79).
- Eat more fish (see page 99).
- Quit smoking (see page 47).

◆

Q: What medications are used to lower triglycerides?
A: Your doctor can prescribe a variety of medications—nicotinic acid, fibrates, statins, and bile acid binders—

that can help reduce your triglyceride levels and improve other blood fats in your lipid profile. These medications are discussed in detail below.

Q: Which of these medications is most often used to lower triglyceride levels?

A: The most popular drug for reducing triglyceride levels is actually a megadose of vitamin B_3 called nicotinic acid (various brand names). If you and your doctor decide to use medication as part of your plan to lower your triglycerides, nicotinic acid may very well be your first choice. You can think of this drug, which is also called niacin, as the "full-court press" of lipid-lowering medications. This one drug can help to lower your LDL cholesterol and triglyceride levels by 10% to 20% while increasing your HDL cholesterol. It works by slowing the production of VLDL in the liver. Nicotinic acid may also reduce levels of fibrinogen, a clotting agent in the blood. As you saw in Chapter 2, a blood clot in an artery is what causes a heart attack or stroke. Nicotinic acid is also effective at decreasing levels of chylomicron remnants in your blood after a meal. In as little as one or two weeks nicotinic acid can begin to change your blood fat levels. Nicotinic acid is relatively inexpensive, and because it is a vitamin, you do not need a prescription to buy it. But this should not become an excuse to "play doctor" and prescribe nicotinic acid for yourself without medical supervision. Americans often view vitamins as something akin to candy. They are actually drugs that can have serious and unwanted side effects at high dosages.

Your doctor may recommend 1½ to 3 g of nicotinic acid three times a day to help lower your triglycerides and change the levels of other fats in your blood (up to 6 g a day is not unheard of). Your doctor will recommend that you start out by taking a small amount of the drug so that your body can adjust to the medication. Then your doctor will gradually increase the dosage to recommended levels. Nicotinic acid may cause flushing or hot flashes—this is a fairly common side effect of medications that dilate (widen) blood vessels. A hot flash is a sudden rush of warmth, lasting anywhere from several seconds to several minutes and varying in intensity, starting in the chest and radiates into the neck and face. Taking nicotinic acid with food can help to alleviate this side effect until your body develops a tolerance to the drug and the hot flashes subside on their own. Nicotinic acid can cause gastrointestinal (GI) effects such as nausea, stomach upset, gas, and diarrhea. The drug may also worsen stomach ulcers and increase your risk of liver problems or gout—the higher the dosage, the higher the risk. Nicotinic acid may enhance the effects of blood pressure–lowering medication, so you should be sure to inform your doctor if you are taking a medication for high blood pressure (or any other drugs). If you have diabetes, your doctor may not recommend nicotinic acid because it raises glucose levels, though there is still some controversy in the medical community regarding the use of nicotinic acid in people with diabetes.

◆

Getting the Most Out of Your Medication

No one cares more about your health than you do. So when your doctor recommends medication as part of a strategy to lower your triglycerides, you owe it to yourself to play an active role in this decision. Always educate yourself about medications before you start taking them, and make sure that you have a clear understanding of why your doctor believes that drugs are necessary. Getting the most out of your medication also means remembering to take it.

Do You Really Need Medication?

Ask your doctor to explain the goals of treatment and how medication will help you to reach those goals. Have you and your doctor exhausted nondrug methods of reducing your triglycerides? As your expert health partner, your doctor should help you to weigh the potential benefits of a drug against its risks.

Know the Side Effects

Ask your doctor about the possible side effects of a medication *before* you start taking it. Most people find it easier to cope with side effects when they know what to expect in advance. Drug reference books are another great source of information. They are available in bookstores and public libraries. Your pharmacist may also be able to provide tips on using your medication safely.

Food or Drug Interactions

Combining your medication with food or other drugs (even those sold over the counter) may alter how it works or lead to unwanted and possibly even dangerous effects. Your doctor should explain whether or not to take your medication with food and should also point out important drug interactions.

Keep a Record

Sometimes it is helpful to make a medication chart for easy reference, especially if you are taking more than one drug at a time. This chart should include basic information about all your medications.

- The names of the drugs
- What they are used for
- When to take them
- Possible side effects
- What to do if you miss a dose
- Whom to call if you have a question about the drugs you are taking or your medication schedule

Remembering to Take Your Medication

This can be more difficult than you think—especially as you get older or if you have a hectic lifestyle. One of the best strategies is to schedule your doses around routine activities. For example, try taking your medication around the same time that you brush your teeth or eat your meals. You can also use your watch alarm or ask friends or family members to assist in helping you remember. If all else fails, the problem may not be you but rather your dosage schedule. Talk to your doctor or pharmacist about simplifying it and making it easier to stick to.

◆

Q: What are fibrates?
A: Fibrate medications such as gemfibrozil (Lopid), clofibrate (Atromid-S), or fenofibrate (Tricor) are effec-

tive at lowering triglycerides and raising HDL cholesterol. Fibrates are not as useful at lowering LDL or total
cholesterol. These drugs lower triglyceride levels by
speeding the rate at which VLDL is removed from the
blood. People who use fibrates may be able to lower their
triglycerides by up to 50% and raise their HDL cholesterol by about 15%. Fibrates are usually taken twice a day
(except for fenofibrate, which is taken once a day) and are
not associated with many bothersome side effects. GI
problems are the most common complaint. These include
stomach upset, nausea, and diarrhea. Fibrates may also
increase the risk of developing gallstones (especially with
long-term use) and enhance the blood-thinning effects of
drugs such as warfarin (Coumadin, Panwarfin, or
Sofarin) or aspirin.

**Q: What are statin drugs and how do they affect
triglyceride levels?**
A: Statins are a shorter name for HMG-CoA reductase
inhibitors. The "HMG-CoA reductase" refers to an
enzyme in the body that helps to regulate the production
of cholesterol. By blocking the action of this enzyme,
HMG-CoA reductase inhibitors can dramatically lower
your cholesterol levels. Unlike nicotinic acid, an HMG-
CoA reductase inhibitor is something of a "specialist"—
and its specialty is being able to lower LDL cholesterol
more than any other drug. Medications in this class have
the power to literally *halve* your LDL cholesterol level
and also significantly reduce your total cholesterol. The
result? People who take HMG-CoA reductase inhibitors
can reduce their risk of CAD and heart attack. Because of
their impressive track record, HMG-CoA reductase
inhibitors are the most frequently prescribed cholesterol-
lowering drugs. You may need the LDL-reducing power
of an HMG-CoA reductase inhibitor if your levels of

LDL cholesterol are high. HMG-CoA reductase inhibitors can also lower your triglycerides, but they are not quite as effective at reducing levels of this fat unless your triglyceride levels are greater than 250 mg/dL.

HMG-CoA reductase inhibitors begin to improve LDL and triglyceride levels within 1 week and at two to three weeks they reach their maximum effect. They are usually taken in single doses at dinner or before going to sleep at night. It is important that these medications be taken in the evening to take advantage of the fact that the body makes more cholesterol at night than during the day. These drugs are not associated with many bothersome side effects in the short term or dangerous drug interactions. GI effects are the most common complaint. These include mild to moderate stomach pain, gas, or cramps as well as constipation—problems that tend to go away with continued use of the medication. We do not know much about the long-term side effects associated with HMG-CoA reductase inhibitors because they have not been studied in people for longer than about five years. A few cautions do apply. Pregnant women should not take HMG-CoA reductase inhibitors because their cholesterol-lowering effects may harm the fetus, which relies on a sufficient amount of cholesterol in order to develop properly. HMG-CoA reductase inhibitors may also pass into breast milk, so nursing mothers who take the medication should bottle-feed their infants with formula and not breast-feed. People with liver disease or those who drink large amounts of alcohol should avoid HMG-CoA reductase inhibitors because these medications may worsen liver problems. In fewer than 1% of people who take HMG-CoA reductase inhibitors, liver or muscle damage may result.

◆

The HMG-CoA Reductase Inhibitors

These drugs have the ability to dramatically lower LDL and total cholesterol levels and to a lesser extent to lower triglyceride and raise HDL levels.

- Atorvastatin (Lipitor)
- Cerivastatin (Baycol)
- Fluvastatin (Lescol)
- Lovastatin (Mevacor)
- Pravastatin (Pravachol)
- Simvastatin (Zocor)

◆

Q: What is a bile acid binder?
A: It is an odd-sounding name for a medication, is it not? Bile acid binders—such as cholestyramine (Prevalite or Questran) and colestipol (Colestid)—are not used alone to lower your triglycerides because they can actually *increase* levels of this blood fat (in some cases these increases are temporary). They are mainly effective at reducing LDL cholesterol in the blood, lowering levels by 10% to 25%. Doctors sometimes combine a bile acid binder with a triglyceride-lowering medication such as nicotinic acid or gemfibrozil in order to lower LDL and total cholesterol while maintaining or decreasing triglycerides. Bile acid binders are so named because of the way they lower cholesterol levels. They do this by attaching themselves to bile acids in your intestine and detouring the bile out of your body via bowel movements.

What is bile and how does it affect cholesterol levels? Bile is a substance made in the liver. It is composed of cholesterol as well as other substances, including bilirubin, the pigment that gives stool its color. Bile helps your body to break down and digest food. When your body is running low on bile—as it is when you take a bile acid binder—it responds by making more of it. In order to do this, the body draws upon the reserves of cholesterol in your blood. The result is lower blood levels of LDL and total cholesterol. If all this sounds a little familiar, it should. As you saw in Chapter 4, fiber is also thought to lower cholesterol levels by interfering with the action of bile and stimulating the body to remove cholesterol from the blood in order to produce sufficient amounts.

Bile acid binders primarily operate in the GI tract and do not circulate in the blood like most lipid-lowering medications. They have been around for about 30 years so doctors are confident about their safety when properly used. In powder form, bile acid binders should be mixed with an adequate amount (about 8 oz.) of water or juice and taken before meals. These side effects include GI problems such as constipation, nausea, gas, and bloating—problems that should ease as you continue to use the medication. Bile acid binders may also worsen hemorrhoids and cause heartburn or appetite loss. They can interfere with the absorption of a variety of other drugs, including over-the-counter medications such as aspirin. Always take other medications at least one hour before or four to six hours after you take a bile acid binder.

Q: Can estrogen medications have an effect on triglycerides?

A: Though we do not have direct proof that lack of estrogen contributes to the development of CAD, we know that the risk of heart disease increases dramatically for women who experience menopause, whether natural or surgical. Most doctors believe that loss of estrogen during menopause is a major reason why postmenopausal women are at increased risk of CAD and heart attack. By connecting to communication ports (called receptors) located on the surfaces of cells, estrogen delivers chemical "messages" that seem to have a healthy effect on most blood-fat levels and the inner surfaces of arteries, where plaque tends to develop. Supplemental estrogen can be used after menopause to help fight heart disease by replacing lost estrogen. Many women also take estrogen to help prevent osteoporosis or control troublesome menopausal symptoms such as hot flashes, night sweats, and vaginal dryness. Estrogen replacement therapy (ERT) consists of estrogen alone, while hormone replacement therapy (HRT) is a combination of estrogen and progestin (a synthetic version of another important female hormone called progesterone). Estrogen therapy can reduce the risk of heart disease by as much as 50% in postmenopausal women. But while estrogen tends to lower LDL cholesterol and raise HDL cholesterol levels, it also tends to raise your triglyceride levels—whether in the form of postmenopausal estrogen therapy or oral contraceptives ("the pill"). If you have elevated triglycerides and are considering using ERT or HRT to help fight heart disease, you and your doctor must carefully weigh the benefits of estrogen against the risk that it will raise your triglyceride levels even further. Estrogen medications are also associated with an increased risk of breast cancer and potentially dangerous blood clots. Selective estrogen receptor modulator (SERM) medications such as raloxifene (Evista)—which may also help to prevent heart disease in postmenopausal women by mimicking the effects of estrogen—may have the same triglyceride-boosting effects as estrogen.

Glossary

adrenal glands: glands located near the kidneys that produce hormones regulating metabolism and blood pressure.

aerobic exercise: any exercise that helps to condition the heart and lungs by making them work harder to meet the increased oxygen demands of the body.

ambulatory electrocardiography: *see* Holter monitor.

amino acid: a building block of protein.

analgesic: pain reliever.

androgen: an important male sex hormone found in small amounts in women.

aneurysm: the "ballooning out" of a section of blood vessel or part of the heart.

angina: chest pain triggered by physical or emotional strain and relieved by rest; angina is associated with coronary artery disease.

angiography: *see* cerebral angiography, coronary angiography

anticoagulant: an agent that prevents coagulation.

antioxidants: a group of vitamins, including vitamins E, C, and beta carotene (a form of vitamin A), that may help to contain free radical damage.

aorta: the artery through which blood leaves the left side of the heart.

aortic stenosis: the narrowing of a valve that leads from the major pumping chamber of the heart, which is called the left ventricle.

aortic valve: the passage between the left ventricle and the aorta.

aphasia: difficulties with speech or comprehension due to a brain injury or disease.

apo-CII: a protein that, along with lipoprotein lipase, aids in removing fatty acids from triglycerides in chylomicrons and very low density lipoprotein; the fatty acids are then used as energy for the body.

arrhythmia: abnormal heartbeat.

arteries: the vessels that carry oxygenated blood away from the heart.

arterioles: small arteries.

aspirin: an over-the-counter pain reliever and anti-inflammatory agent that can help to prevent heart attacks and heart disease.

atherogenic: having the ability to contribute to the development of atherosclerosis.

atherosclerosis: narrowing and hardening of the arteries.

"bad" cholesterol: *see* low-density lipoprotein (LDL) cholesterol.

balloon dilation: a procedure in which a catheter with a balloon at its tip is inserted into an artery in the leg and guided up to the aorta to a narrowed coronary artery in the heart; the balloon is then inflated to widen the narrowed area and increase blood flow in the artery.

beta blockers: a class of medications that help decrease tension in the heart wall, leading to less oxygen consumption, as well as helping to control blood pressure by blocking the activity of substances like epinephrine, a hormone that boosts blood pressure.

bile: an acidic mix of cholesterol, bilirubin (the pigment that gives stool its color), and other substances whose detergent-like action is important in breaking down and digesting food.

blood clot: blood that has coagulated and formed a solid mass.

blood pressure: the force that blood exerts on the walls of the vessels.

blood vessels: flexible tubes that carry blood through the body.

bone density: the amount of mineral in any given volume of bone.

bone density test: a medical test used to measure the strength of the bones.

bradycardia: abnormally slow heartbeat.

CAD: *see* coronary artery disease.

caffeine: a stimulant found in coffee, tea, some sodas, and chocolate.

calcium: a mineral that acts as an important building block of bone and is used by the body for proper functioning of organs and muscles.

cancer: an unrestrained growth of abnormal cells, often in the form of a tumor, that invades and destroys healthy tissue.

capillaries: the tiny vessels that connect arteries with veins.

carbohydrate: compounds of the elements carbon, oxygen, and hydrogen that are related to sugars and foods such as breads, pastas, and potatoes.

carbon monoxide: a noxious gas found in cigarette smoke that damages artery walls and thickens blood.

cardiac: relating to the heart.

cardiac arrest: the stopping of the heartbeat.

cardiologist: a doctor who specializes in treating cardiovascular diseases.

cardiomyopathy: weakening of the heart muscle that results in reduced pumping power.

cardiovascular: relating to the cardiovascular system.

cardiovascular disease: any of a number of disorders that affect the circulatory system.

cardiovascular system: the system composed mainly of the heart and blood vessels that is responsible for circulating blood throughout the body.

carotid arteries: the major arteries in the neck that supply the brain with blood.

catheter: a flexible, hollow tube inserted into various parts of the body to inject or suction out fluids.

cerebral angiography: this procedure is similar to coronary angiography except that it is used to detect atherosclerosis in the main arteries supplying the brain with blood (as opposed to those that serve the heart). See also coronary angiography.

cerebral hemorrhage: bleeding into the brain.

cerebrovascular: relating to blood vessels in the brain.

cholesterol: a waxy substance made by the body and found in foods that come from animals; cholesterol is the main ingredient of plaque. Cholesterol is a substance that does not dissolve in water and is greasy to the touch.

cholestyramine: a medication used to lower low-density lipoprotein cholesterol by reducing the amount of bile acid available to make cholesterol.

chylomicron: a tiny, spherical particle composed of triglyceride, cholesterol, and protein released in large numbers into the bloodstream following a meal.

chylomicron remnant: a smaller, cholesterol-rich particle that results from chylomicron processing in the bloodstream.

circulatory system: the system composed mainly of the heart and blood vessels that provides oxygen and nutrients to all parts of the body.

claudication: pain or weakness in the extremities due to decreased oxygen supply in the muscles.

clofibrate (Atromid-S): a medication that is used to help the body reduce the level of triglycerides in the blood.

coagulation: the process of changing blood from a liquid to a semisolid or solid, typically through the action of clotting proteins.

collateral blood vessels: tiny blood vessels that enlarge in some people with coronary artery disease in order to reroute blood flow around plaque deposits in arteries.

colon: the tube connecting the small intestine with the anus.

congenital: present at birth.

congestive heart failure: a condition in which the heart is unable to pump enough blood to serve the needs of the body.

coronary angiography: a procedure that involves injecting a radioactive dye into the coronary arteries and taking moving X ray images.

coronary arteries: the arteries that supply the heart muscle with blood.

coronary artery bypass surgery: a procedure that improves blood flow to heart muscle by removing a blood vessel from another part of the body and using it to bypass a severely clogged coronary artery.

coronary artery disease (CAD): a condition characterized by reduced blood flow to the heart due to narrowing and hardening of the coronary arteries.

coronary artery spasm: involuntary muscle contractions of a coronary artery.

coronary circulation: the vessel by which blood pumped by the heart is sent right back to the organ to provide oxygen and nutrients to the heart.

coronary occlusion: an obstruction in a coronary artery that reduces blood flow to the heart.

coronary thrombosis: the formation of a clot in one of the arteries that carry blood to the heart muscle.

cyanosis: low oxygen levels in the blood.

defibrillator: a machine used by doctors or emergency service workers to restore heartbeat.

deoxygenated blood: bluish blood containing carbon dioxide waste.

diabetes: a condition characterized by an inability to produce adequate amounts of insulin or to utilize the hormone properly.

diaphragm: a fanlike muscle lying between the chest and abdominal cavities, used for normal breathing.

diastolic: relating to the resting phase of the heartbeat.

diastolic blood pressure: the pressure of the blood when the heart is momentarily resting between beats; it is the second number in the blood pressure measurement.

dietary: derived from food or drink.

digestion: the process of converting food into substances that can be used by the body.

dilate: widen.

diuretics: agents that increase urination.

dyspnea: shortness of breath.

dysrhythmia: an abnormal heart rhythm.

early menopause: menopause that occurs before age 40.

echocardiogram: a procedure that uses sound waves to create an image of the inside of the heart in order to reveal the shape and motion of the heart's four chambers and valves.

edema: swelling (usually of the hands or feet) due to the accumulation of fluid in tissues.

eicosanoids: hormone-like substances that play a role in regulating blood pressure and circulation, preventing blood clots, and keeping the immune system strong.

electrocardiogram (ECG or EKG): a recording that represents a graphic representation of the heartbeat in order to assess heart muscle damage or enlargement as well as abnormal heart rhythms such as arrhythmias or dysrhythmias.

embolus: a moving blood clot.

endocarditis: a bacterial infection of the endocardium, typically associated with a valve.

endocardium: the membrane that lines the inside surface of the heart.

endocrine system: a complex biological network composed of organs and glands that secrete hormones to other areas of the body in order to regulate reproduction and growth, digestion, bone building, calorie burning, body temperature, and metabolism.

enzyme: a protein found in cells and digestive juices that stimulates chemical reactions in the body.

epithelium: the layer of cells covering surfaces of the body such as the skin or internal tubes or cavities.

esophagus: the tube connecting the mouth to the stomach.

essential fatty acids: any acid that occurs naturally in fats that cannot be produced by the human body and must be obtained from food.

estradiol: the main form of estrogen produced by the ovaries.

estrogen: the primary female sex hormone; estrogen helps to keep the cardiovascular system healthy and prevent heart disease in women.

estrogen receptors: proteins on the surfaces of cells that bind with estrogen.

estrogen replacement therapy (ERT): the use of an estrogen medication to raise levels of the hormone following menopause.

excrete: to eliminate or remove.

exercise stress test: a procedure used to evaluate heart function that involves walking or jogging on a treadmill or pedaling a stationary bike.

familial combined hyperlipidemia (FCH): an inherited condition in which members of the same family have high cholesterol and/or triglycerides and tend to develop heart disease early in life (before age 55). FCH is associated with increased production of very low density lipoprotein cholesterol in the liver.

familial hypertriglyceridemia (FHT): a blood fat disorder that runs in families. FHT occurs when the liver produces a normal amount of very low-density lipoprotein but the particles are too large. High levels of triglyceride and very low-density lipoprotein are accompanied by a normal amount of low-density lipoprotein cholesterol.

fatty acid: a building block of fat.

fiber: indigestible substances found in fruits, vegetables, grains, and nuts.

fibrin: an insoluble protein that acts as a clotting agent in the blood.

flutter: irregular contractions of the heart muscle.

free radicals: molecular fragments of oxygen produced as a byproduct when cells use oxygen to burn fat; free radicals roam through the body causing damage to cells and to genes that regulate how cells grow.

gemfibrozil (Lopid): a medication used to lower triglyceride levels due to its ability to decrease very low-density lipoprotein levels.

gland: a cell (or group of cells) or an organ that produces substances (such as hormones) used by the body.

glucose: blood sugar.

good cholesterol: *see* high-density lipoprotein (HDL) cholesterol.

HDL: *see* high-density lipoprotein (HDL) cholesterol.

heart: the powerful dual pump that circulates blood to all the organs and tissues in the body and removes waste products such as carbon dioxide.

heart attack: a cardiac event that occurs when the blood supply to part of the heart muscle is obstructed or severely reduced due to a blood clot that forms near an eruption of atherosclerotic plaque; also called myocardial infarction.

heartbeat: the sound made by the operation of the valves during a full heart cycle.

heart block: an interruption of the electrical impulses that make the heart beat.

hemoglobin: a protein in red blood cells that gives blood its red color and acts as a magnet for both oxygen and carbon dioxide.

hemorrhage: bleeding.

high-density lipoprotein (HDL) cholesterol: a particle that transports cholesterol away from the arteries and back to the liver, where it is eliminated or transformed into other substances needed by the body; also called "good" cholesterol.

Holter monitor: a small, battery-powered ECG unit that can be worn for one or two days while it records the electrical activity of the heart; also called ambulatory electrocardiography.

hormone: a chemical message carrier produced by an organ or gland that travels through the bloodstream to specific receptors located on the cells of other organs or glands.

hormone receptors: "communication ports" located on the surfaces of cells that allow hormones like estrogen to deliver chemical messages to cells.

hormone replacement therapy (HRT): the use of an estrogen-progesterone medication to raise levels of estrogen after menopause.

hot flash: a sudden rush of warmth, lasting anywhere from several seconds to several minutes and varying in intensity, that starts in the chest and radiates into the neck and face.

hydrogenated fat: fat that has become more saturated after undergoing a manufacturing process called hydrogenation.

hydrogenation: a food-manufacturing process that involves bombarding heart-healthy polyunsaturated fatty acids (such as those found in vegetable oil) with hydrogen ions in order to enhance the shelf life of a product or thicken its consistency.

hyperplasia: excessive cell growth.

hypertension: high blood pressure.

hypoglycemia: low blood sugar.

hypothalamus: the part of the brain above the pituitary gland that regulates many body functions such as body temperature, sleep, and appetite.

hypothyroidism: underactive thyroid gland.

hysterectomy: a surgical procedure in which the entire uterus is removed.

ideal weight: the amount that you are expected to weigh based on variables such as gender and height.

insulin: a hormone produced by the pancreas that helps the body to use sugar.

invasive: a procedure that involves puncturing the skin or the insertion of an instrument into the body.

ischemia: inadequate oxygenation of tissue due to reduced blood flow to an organ typically from arterial blockage.

jugular vein: one of the vessels that carry blood from the head back to the heart.

larynx: voice box.

LDL cholesterol: *see* low-density lipoprotein (LDL) cholesterol.

left atrium: the filling chamber above the left ventricle that receives blood returning from the lungs.

left ventricle: the powerful pump on the left side of the heart that forces newly oxygenated blood out of the heart and into all the tissues and organs of the body.

lesion: a wound or injury.

lipid: a triglyceride or cholesterol in the blood.

lipoprotein: a type of protein that transports lipids in the blood.

lipoprotein lipase: a protein in the blood that helps to break down chylomicrons and very low-density lipoprotein by stripping them of fatty acids.

low-density lipoprotein (LDL) cholesterol: A cholesterol-carrying particle that tends to dump its cargo of fat onto artery linings, where it can accumulate and form plaque; also called "bad" cholesterol. It is measured by the amount of cholesterol in the particle.

lymphatic system: a system of organs and tissues that is vital to the body's ability to fight infection and disease.

lymph vessels: tiny tubes, branching into all the tissues of the body, that collect the fluid circulating between cells and transport it to the lymph nodes for filtering.

mechanism of action: the process or processes by which a medication produces its effects.

menopause: the day on which menstrual periods have stopped for one year, occurring around age 50; the term is also used to refer to the entire process during which the ovaries slow down and finally cease producing estrogen.

mineral: an inorganic substance necessary in small amounts for good health and proper functioning of the body.

mini-stroke: *see* transient ischemic attack.

mitral valve: the valve that connects the left atrium to the left ventricle.

monounsaturated fat: a dietary fat, found in olive and canola oil as well as in avocados that many propose should replace saturated fat in our diet and that generally does not affect the levels of high density lipoprotein.

mutate: change.

myocardial infarction: *see* heart attack.

myocardium: the layer of cardiac muscle that covers the outer portion of the heart.

necrosis: tissue death.

nicotine: a chemical found in cigarette smoke that encourages the buildup of plaque in arteries.

night sweats: hot flashes that occur at night during sleep.

nitroglycerin: a medication that dilates the arteries.

noninvasive: nonpenetrating; a procedure that does not involve puncturing the skin or inserting an instrument into the body.

obesity: an excess of body fat that equals 20% or more of a person's ideal weight.

olestra: a fat replacer sometimes used by food manufacturers in place of other fats in order to create a fat-free or low-fat product with the same texture and taste of foods fried in regular oil.

omega-3: an essential fatty acid found primarily in fish, green leafy vegetables, nuts, and soybeans.

omega-6: an essential fatty acid found primarily in fish, green leafy vegetables, grains, and seeds.

oophorectomy: the surgical removal of the ovaries.

osteoporosis: an age-related, gradual weakening of the bones that causes them to become more fragile and vulnerable to potentially debilitating fractures.

ovary: the female reproductive organ that produces eggs; the ovaries are where most estrogen is made in women.

oxygenated blood: bright red blood laden with oxygen.

palpate: to feel.

palpitation: irregular heartbeat.

pancreas: an organ situated behind the stomach that produces digestive enzymes and the hormone insulin.

pancreatitis: an inflammation of the pancreas that can occur as a result of very high triglyceride levels.

pericarditis: an inflammation of the pericardium.

pericardium: a thin, translucent sac that surrounds the outside of the heart and protects the organ from invasion by infections from other parts of the body such as the lungs.

placebo: a sugar pill.

plaque: a deposit of cholesterol and other substances that thickens the walls of an artery and forces blood to squeeze through a narrower than normal space.

plasma: a clear, yellowish liquid made mostly of water that accounts for about half of blood; plasma transports most of the substances in the blood.

platelets: "sticky," irregularly shaped cells in the blood that routinely rush to the scene of an injury or wound and clump together to help seal off the injured area and stop the bleeding.

polyunsaturated fat: a dietary fat, found in many cooking oils (including sunflower and sesame oil) and in margarine. It is often used as a replacement for saturated fats.

postmenopausal: a term referring to a woman who has completed menopause.

postprandial: after a meal.

progesterone: an important female sex hormone, made by the ovaries, that helps to prepare the uterus for the fertilized egg and for the growth of the fetus.

progestin: a synthetic version of progesterone.

prognosis: the outlook for recovery.

prolapse: a condition in which part of the body moves out of its normal position.

protein: a substance made up of amino acids that helps to grow and repair tissue in the body.

pulmonary: relating to the lungs.

pulmonary circulation: the process by which bluish, deoxygenated blood is pumped through the lungs in order to exchange carbon dioxide for oxygen.

pulmonary edema: severe accumulation of fluid in the lungs.

pulmonary embolism: a blood clot in the arteries of the lungs.

pulmonic valve: the valve that regulates the flow of blood from the right side of the heart into the artery leading to the lungs.

radiation: a type of energy found in X rays and ultraviolet light.

red blood cells: the cells that deliver oxygen to tissues and remove carbon dioxide and other waste.

regurgitation: backward flow of blood due to an improperly working valve in the heart.

renal: relating to the kidneys.

respiration: the act of breathing.

right atrium: the filling chamber above the right ventricle that receives old blood returning from its round trip through the body.

right ventricle: the low-pressure pump on the right side of the heart that propels old, deoxygenated blood along its short circuit through the lungs.

risk factor: anything that increases the likelihood of developing a particular disease.

saturated fat: a dietary fat, found in foods that come from animals as well as certain oils, that can raise cholesterol levels more than anything else in the diet.

selective estrogen receptor modulator: a type of medication that mimics the effects of estrogen in certain parts of the body while blocking its effects in others.

septal defect: a hole in the wall of muscle that separates the right from the left side of the heart.

septum: the wall of muscle that separates the left and right sides of the heart.

serotonin: a hormone that in proper amounts can help to control appetite and produce a sense of emotional well-being.

serum: the fluid that remains after platelets and other clotting agents are removed from the blood.

signal average electrocardiogram: a type of electrocardiogram that records more information than a standard electrocardiogram and takes longer to conduct. It is used to predict a predisposition to life-threatening arrythmias.

sinus node: an area of tissue in the right filling chamber that generates the electrical charge that starts the heartbeat.

sonogram: an image produced by sound waves.

sonography: the use of high-frequency sound waves to create an image of the inside of the body.

sphygmomanometer: an instrument used to measure blood pressure.

stenosis: the narrowing of a duct or canal in the body.

sternum: breastbone.

stethoscope: an instrument primarily used to listen to heartbeat.

stress: physical or emotional strain.

stroke: damage to brain cells due to lack of blood supply; usually caused by either an obstructed artery or an artery that bursts and bleeds into surrounding tissue, a stroke leaves brain cells in the affected area starved for oxygen and unable to function.

surgical menopause: an onset of menopause caused by the surgical removal of the ovaries.

systemic: referring to the whole body.

systemic circulation: the process by which fresh, oxygenated blood is pumped by the heart through an extensive network of blood vessels that reaches into every corner of the body.

systolic: relating to the beating phase of the heartbeat.

systolic blood pressure: the pressure of blood in the arteries when the heart muscles are contracting during a heartbeat; it is the first number in the blood pressure measurement.

tachycardia: rapid heartbeat.

tachypnea: rapid breathing.

testosterone: a male sex hormone produced in the testes.

thallium stress test: a procedure that evaluates the flow of blood to the heart by combining an exercise stress test with a dye-enhanced imaging procedure.

thrombus: a stationary blood clot.

TIA: *see* transient ischemic attack (TIA).

tilt table test: a procedure that involves moving the body through various angles in order to determine if a person is vulnerable to sudden changes in blood pressure or pulse rate.

tissue: a mass of cells.

total cholesterol: the total amount of cholesterol in a standard unit of blood, typically 1 milliliter.

transesophageal echocardiogram (TEE): an invasive procedure that involves placing a transducer, a device that measures sound waves, close to the heart by inserting it into the esophagus to obtain a clear image of the heart.

trans fatty acids: a special breed of fatty acid, present in most stick margarines and other foods made with hydrogenated oil at high temperatures, that can modestly change total cholesterol levels and lower high-density lipoprotein levels. Trans fatty acids are associated with atherosclerosis.

transient ischemic attack (TIA): a strokelike event whose symptoms last only a few minutes to a half hour; also called a ministroke.

tricuspid valve: the valve that connects the right atrium to the right ventricle.

triglycerides: the form in which most dietary and body fat exists; the term is also used to refer to the total amount of triglyceride in the blood.

tropical oils: a group of oils high in saturated fat that includes coconut oil, palm kernel oil, and palm oil.

unsaturated fat: a type of fat that may have a healthy effect on the heart when used in moderation.

valve: a membranous fold in a canal or passage that ensures the one-way flow of the contents passing through it.

valvuloplasty: surgery designed to repair a defective or improperly working heart valve.

variant angina: a type of chest pain that occurs at rest and is associated with coronary artery spasm; also called Prinzmetal's angina.

varicose vein: an abnormally dilated vein.

vascular: relating to blood vessels.

vasculitis: an inflammation of a blood vessel.

vasoconstriction: narrowing of a blood vessel.

vasodilator: a medication, or natural body substance, that dilates blood vessels.

veins: the vessels that carry deoxygenated blood back to the heart.

vena cava: the two large veins through which blood enters the right side of the heart.

ventricle: one of the two pumps located in the lower half of the heart.

very low-density lipoprotein (VLDL): a lipoprotein that primarily transports triglycerides along with a small amount of cholesterol; it is typically measured by its cholesterol content.

very low-density lipoprotein (VLDL) remnant: a smaller, cholesterol-rich type of low-density lipoprotein.

vitamin: an organic substance necessary in small amounts for good health and proper functioning of the body.

VLDL: *see* very low-density lipoprotein (VLDL).

weight-bearing exercise: any exercise that builds muscle and strengthens bone.

white blood cells: the cells that seek and destroy disease-causing microorganisms that invade the body.

xanthomas: deposits of cholesterol and triglyceride that may be visible under the skin, appearing as reddish-yellow streaks or bumps on the arms or legs.

X ray: an image of the inside of the body produced by a machine that emits small amounts of radiation.

Bibliography and Further Reading

Going to the Source

What can a layperson learn from a medical study? Probably more than you think. Though you can play an active role in your health care without looking at articles from professional medical journals, these studies are a great resource for those who wish to go directly to the source instead of relying on newspaper columns and TV reports to interpret health-related research. It is in the pages of the top medical journals that doctors examine some of the most important questions regarding triglycerides:

- How do elevated triglycerides affect middle-aged men or postmenopausal women?
- Why do doctors now believe that the tiny balls of fat called chylomicron remnants can deposit cholesterol onto artery walls?
- How effective is the medication I'm taking to lower my triglyceride levels?

With a medical dictionary and a little patience, you may find that you can listen in to the ongoing scientific dialogue concerning these and other questions about triglycerides and their role in the development of coronary artery disease (CAD). Medical studies also continue to shed new light on the process of atherosclerosis (the narrowing and hardening of the arteries) and on risk factors for heart disease. By looking at some of this research you can familiarize yourself with important medical terms in context and have more productive discussions with your doctor about your care. If you have access to the Internet, many medical studies are available in summary form via an online service called MEDLINE. With the push of a button you can use this free, searchable database containing thousands of medical-journal abstracts. You may be able to see these articles in their complete form by searching the Internet or going to your local library or that of a medical school in your area. It is also important to remember that not all medical studies present the same degree of difficulty. Articles that investigate triglycerides or the process of atherosclerosis on a microscopic level are some of the most interesting but are usually expressed in more technical language than those that examine groups of people.

Alaupovic P., Heinonen T., Shurzinske L., et al. Effect of a new HMG-CoA reductase inhibitor, atorvastatin, on lipids, apolipoproteins and lipoprotein particles in patients with elevated serum cholesterol and triglyceride levels. *Atherosclerosis* 1997; 133:123–133.

Alaupovic P., Mack W. J., Knight-Gibson C., et al. The role of triglyceride-rich lipoprotein families in the progress of atherosclerotic lesions are determined by sequential coronary angiography from a controlled clinical trial. *Arterioscler Thromb Vasc Biol* 1997; 17:715–722.

Albrink M. J. and Man E. B. Serum triglycerides in coronary artery disease. *Arch Int Med* 1959; 103:4–8.

American College of Physicians. Guidelines for using serum cholesterol, high-density lipoprotein cholesterol, and triglyceride levels as screening tests for preventing coronary heart disease in adults. *Ann Intern Med* 1996; 124:515–517.

American Dietetic Association. http://www.eatright.org

American Heart Association. http://www.amhrt.org

American Medical Association. http://www.ama-assn.org

Annuzzi G., Rivellese A., Capaldo B., et al. A controlled study on the effects of n-3 fatty acids on lipid and glucose metabolism in non-insulin-dependent diabetic patients. *Atherosclerosis* 1991; 87:65–73.

Ashbourne Excoffon K. J. D., Liu G., Miao L., et al. Correction of hypertriglyceridemia and impaired fat tolerance in lipoprotein lipase-deficient mice by adenovirus-mediated expression of human lipoprotein lipase. *Arterioscler Thromb Vasc Biol* 1997; 17:2532–2539.

Assmann G. and Schulte H. Relation of high-density lipoprotein cholesterol and triglycerides to incidence of atherosclerotic coronary artery disease (the PRO-CAM experience). Prospective Cardiovascular Munster Study. *Am J Cardiol* 1992; 70:733–7.

Assmann G., Schulte H., and von Eckardstein A. Hypertriglyceridemia and elevated lipoprotein(a) are risk factors for major coronary events in middle-aged men. *Am J Cardiol* 1996; 77:1179–1184.

Attwood C. R. Low-fat diets for children: practicality and safety. *Am J Cardiol* 1998; 82:77–79.

Auerback O., Carter H. W., Garfinkel L., et al. Cigarette smoking and coronary artery disease: a macroscopic and microscopic study. *Chest* 1976; 70:697–705.

Austin M. A. Genetic epidemiology of dyslipidaemia and atherosclerosis. *Ann Med* 1996; 28:459–463.

Austin M. A. Triacylglycerol and coronary heart disease. *Proc Nutr Soc* 1997; 56: 667–670.

Austin M. A. Plasma triglyceride and coronary heart disease. *Arterioscler Thromb* 1991; 11:2–14.

Austin M. A. and Hokanson J.E. Epidemiology of triglycerides, small dense low-density lipoprotein, and lipoprotein(a) as risk factors for coronary heart disease. *Med Clin North Am* 1994; 78:99–115.

Austin M. A., Hokanson J. E., Edwards K.L. Hyper-triglyceridemia as a cardiovascular risk factor. *Am J. Cardiol* 1998; 81(4A): 7B–12B.

Bagdade J. D., Buchanan W. E., Levy R. A., et al. Effects of n-3 fish oils on plasma lipids, lipoprotein composition and postheparin lipoprotein lipase in women with NIDDM. *Diabetes* 1990; 30:426–31.

Bainton D., Miller N. E., Bolton C. H., et al. Plasma triglyceride and high-density lipoprotein cholesterol as predictors of ischaemic heart disease in British men: The Caerphilly and Speedwell Collaborative Heart Disease Studies. *Br Heart J* 1992; 68:60–66.

Bakker-Arkema R. G., Davidson M. H., Goldstein R. J., et al. Efficacy and safety of a new HMG-CoA reductase inhibitor, atorvastatin, in patients with hyper-triglyceridemia. *JAMA* 1996; 275:128–133.

Bhatnagar D., Durrington P. N., Mackness M. I., et al. Effects of treatment of hypertriglyceridaemia with gemfibrozil on serum lipoproteins and the transfer of cholesteryl ester from high density lipoproteins to low density lipoproteins. *Atherosclerosis* 1992; 92:49–57.

Bierman E. L. Atherogenesis in diabetes. *Arterioscler Thromb* 1992; 12:647–56.

Boquist S., Ruotolo G., Hellénius M., et al. Effects of a cardioselective blocker on postprandial triglyceride-rich lipoproteins, low density lipoprotein particle size and glucose-insulin homeostasis in middle-aged men with modestly increased cardiovascular risk. *Atherosclerosis* 1998; 137:391–400.

Braunwald E., ed. Heart disease: A textbook of cardiovascular medicine. 3rd ed. 1988; Philadelphia: W. B. Saunders Company.

Breslow J. L. Mouse models of atherosclerosis. *Science* 1996; 272:685–8.

Brischetto C. S., Connor W. E., and Conner S. L. Plasma lipid and lipoprotein profiles of cigarette smokers from randomly selected families. Enhancement of hyperlipidemia and depression of high density lipoprotein. *Am J Cardiol* 1983; 52:675–80.

Brown G., Albers J. J., Fisher L. D., et al. Regression of coronary artery disease as a result of intensive lipid-lowering therapy in men with high levels of apolipoprotein B. *N Engl J Med* 1990; 323:1289–1298.

Brown M. S. and Goldstein J. L. A receptor-mediated pathway for cholesterol homeostasis. *Science* 1986; 232:34–47.

Buchwald H., Varco R. L., Matts J. P., et al. Effect of partial ileal bypass surgery on mortality and morbidity from coronary heart disease in patients with hypercholesterolaemia. Report of the Program on the Surgical Control of Hyperlipidaemia (POSCH). *New Engl J Med* 1990; 323:946–955.

Burr M. L., Gilbert J. F., Holliday R. M., et al. Effects of changes in fat, fish and fibre intakes on death and myocardial reinfarction: diet and reinfarction trial (DART) *Lancet* 1989; 1:757–761.

Carlson L. A. and Böttiger L. E. Ischaemic heart disease in relation to fasting values of plasma triglycerides and cholesterol. Stockholm Prospective Study. *Lancet* 1972; 1:865–868.

Carlson L. A. and Rosenhamer G. Reduction in mortality in the Stockholm Ischaemic Heart Disease Secondary

Prevention Study by combined treatment with clofibrate and nicotinic acid. *Acta Med Scand* 1988; 223:405–18.

Castelli W.P. Epidemiology of triglycerides: A view from Framingham. *Am J Cardiol* 1992; 70:3H–9H.

Chait A., Brazg R., Tribble D., et al. Susceptibility of small, dense, low-density lipoproteins to oxidative modification in subjects with the atherogenic lipoprotein phenotype, pattern B. *Am J Med* 1993; 94:350–356.

Channon K. M., Clegg R. J., Bhatnagar D., et al. Investigation of lipid transfer in human serum leading to the development of an isotopic method for the determination of endogenous cholesterol esterification and transfer. *Atherosclerosis* 1990; 80:217–226.

Collins R., Peto R., MacMahon S., et al. Blood pressure, stroke and coronary heart disease. Part 2. Short-term reductions in blood pressure: Overview of randomised drug trials in their epidemiological context. *Lancet* 1990; 335:827–38.

Conroy R.M., Mulcahy R., Hickey N., et al. Is family history of coronary heart disease an independent coronary risk factor? *Br Heart J* 1985; 53:378–81.

Coronary Drug Project Research Group. Clofibrate and niacin in coronary heart disease. *JAMA* 1975; 231:360–381.

Dart A., Sherrard B., and Simpson H. Influence of apo E phenotype on postprandial triglyceride and glucose responses in subjects with and without coronary heart disease. *Atherosclerosis* 1997; 130:161–170.

Daugherty A., Lange L. G., Sobel B.E., et al. Aortic accumulation and plasma clearance of beta-VLDL and HDL: Effects of diet-induced hypercholesterolemia in rabbits. *J Lipid Res* 1985; 26:955–63.

de Baker G., Kornitzer M., Kittel F., et al. Behavior, stress, and pyschosocial traits as risk factors. *Prev Med* 1983; 12:32–6.

De Graaf J., Hak-Lemmers H., Hectors M., et al. Enhanced susceptibility to in vitro oxidation of the dense low-density lipoprotein sub-fraction in healthy subjects. *Arterioscler Thromb* 1991; 11:298–306.

DeFronzo R. A. and Ferrannini E. Insulin resistance: a multifaceted syndrome responsible for NIDDM, obesity, hypertension, dyslipidemia and atherosclerotic cardiovascular disease. *Diabetes Care* 1991; 14:173–94.

de Lorgeril M., Salen P., Martin J. L. et al. Mediterranean diet, traditional risk factors, and the rate of cardiovascular complications after myocardial infarction: final report of the Lyon Diet Heart Study. *Circulation* 1999; 99:779–785.

Demacker P., Bredie S., Vogelaar J., et al. VLDL accumulation in familial dysbetalipoproteinemia is associated with increased exchange or diffusion of chylomicron lipids to apo B-100 containing triglyceride-rich lipoproteins. *Atherosclerosis* 1998; 138:301–312.

Despres J. P., Lamarche B., Mauriege P., et al. Hyperinsulinemia as an independent risk factor for ischemic heart disease. *N Engl J Med* 1996; 334:952–7.

Durrington P. N. Biological variation in serum lipid concentrations. *Scand J Clin Lab Investig* 1990; 50:86–91.

Durrington P. N. Hyperlipidaemia. *Diagnosis and Management*. 2nd Ed. Oxford: Butterworth-Heinemann, 1995.

Durrington P. N. Triglycerides are more important in atherosclerosis than epidemiology has suggested. *Atherosclerosis* 1998; 141:57–62.

Ehsani A. A., Martin W.H., Heath G.W., et al. Cardiac effects of prolonged and intense exercise training in patients with coronary artery disease. *Am J Cardiol* 1982; 50:246–54.

Endres S., De Caterina R., Schmidt E. B., et al. N-3 Polyunsaturated fatty acids: Update 1995. *Eur J Clin Invest* 1995; 25:629–38.

Ericsson C.-G., Hamsten A., Nilsson J., et al. Angiographic assessment of effects of bezafibrate on progression of coronary artery disease in young male post-infarction patients. *Lancet* 1996; 347:849–853.

Eriksson P., Nilsson L., Karpe F., et al. Very-low-density lipoprotein response element in the promoter region of the human plasminogen activator inhibitor-1 gene implicated in the impaired fibrinolysis of hypertriglyceridemia. *Arterioscler Thromb Vasc Biol* 1998; 18:20–26.

Eritsland J., Deljeflot I., Abdelnoor M., et al. Long-term effects of n-3 fatty acids on serum lipids and glycaemic control. *Scand J Clin Lab Invest* 1994; 54:273–80.

Fontbonne A., Eschwege E., Cambien F., et al. Hypertriglyceridaemia as a risk factor of coronary heart disease mortality in subjects with impaired glucose tolerance or diabetes. Results from the 11-year follow-up of the Paris Prospective Study. *Diabetologia* 1989; 32:300–304.

Food and Drug Administration. http://www.fda.gov

Fraser G. E., Anderson J. T., Foster N., et al. The effect of alcohol on serum high density lipoproteins. *Atherosclerosis* 1983; 46:275–86.

Fredrickson D. S., Morganroth J., and Levy B. I. Type III hyperlipoproteinemia. *Ann Intern Med* 1975; 82:150–157.

Frick M. H., Elo O., Haapa K., et al. Helsinki Heart Study: Primary-prevention trial with gemfibrozil in middle-aged men with dyslipidaemia. Safety of treatment, changes in risk factors, and incidence of coronary heart disease. *New Engl J Med* 1987; 317:1237–1245.

Frick M. H., Syvänne M., Nieminen M. S., et al. Prevention of the angiographic progression of coronary and vein-graft atherosclerosis by gemfibrozil after coronary bypass surgery in men with low levels of HDL cholesterol. *Circulation* 1997; 96:2137–2143.

Friday K. E., Childs M. T., Tsunehara C. H., et al. Elevated plasma glucose and lowered triglyceride levels from omega-3 fatty acid supplementation in type II diabetes. *Diabetes Care* 1989; 12:276–81.

Galeano N. F., Milne R., Marcel Y. L., et al. Apoprotein B structure and receptor recognition of triglyceride-rich low density lipoprotein (LDL) is modified in small LDL but not in triglyceride-rich LDL of normal size. *J Biol Chem* 1994; 269:511–519.

Galli C., Tremoli E., Stragliotto E., et al. Treatment with omega-3 fatty acid ethyl esters in hyperlipoproteinemias: comparative studies on lipid metabolism and thrombotic indexes. *Pharmacol Res* 1995; 31:1–8.

Garrison R. J., Kannel W. B., Feinleib M., et al. Cigarette smoking and HDL cholesterol: The Framingham offspring study. *Atherosclerosis* 1978; 30:17–25.

Gaw A., Packard C. J., Caslake M. J., et al. Effects of ciprofibrate on LDL metabolism in man. *Atherosclerosis* 1994; 108:137–148.

Gianturco S. H., Ramprasad M. P., Lin A. H., et al. Cellular binding site and membrane binding proteins for triglyceride-rich lipoproteins in human monocyte-macrophages and THP-1 monocytic cells. *J Lipid Res* 1994; 35:1674–1687.

Ginsberg H. N. Is hypertriglyceridemia a risk factor for atherosclerotic cardiovascular disease? A simple question with a complicated answer. *Ann Intern Med* 1997; 126:912–914.

Ginsberg H. N. Lipoprotein metabolism and its relationship to atherosclerosis. *Med Clin North Am* 1994; 78:1–20.

Ginsberg H. N., Jones J., Blaner W. S., et al. Association of postprandial triglyceride and retinyl palmitate responses with newly diagnosed exercise-induced myocardial ischemia in middle-aged men and women. *Arterioscler Thromb Vasc Biol* 1995; 15:1829–38.

Gofman J. W., de Lalla O., Glazier F., et al. The serum lipoprotein transport system in health, metabolic disorders, atherosclerosis and coronary artery disease. *Plasma* 1954; 2:413–484.

Goldstein J. L., Hazzard W. R., Schrott H. G., et al. Hyperlipidaemia in coronary heart disease 1. Lipid levels in 500 survivors of myocardial infarction. *J Clin Investig* 1973; 52:1533–1543.

Gordon T., Castelli W. P., Hjortland, M. C., et al. High density lipoprotein as a protective factor against coronary heart disease. The Framingham Study. *Am J Med* 1977; 62:707–714.

Gordon T., Kannel W. B., Hjortland M. C., et al. Menopause and coronary heart disease. The Framingham Study. *Ann Intern Med* 1978; 89:157–61.

Gotto Jr. A. Triglyceride as a risk factor for coronary artery disease. *J Am Cardiol* 1998; 82:22–25.

Grundy S. M. Small LDL, atherogenic dyslipidemia and the metabolic syndrome. *Circulation* 1997; 95:1–4.

Hamsten A. Hypertriglyceridemia, triglyceride-rich lipoproteins and coronary heart disease. *Baillieres Clin Endocrinol Metabol* 1990; 4:895–922.

Harris W. S. Fish oils and plasma lipid and lipoprotein metabolism in humans: A critical review. *J Lipid Res* 1989; 30:785–807.

Haynes S. A., Feinleib M., and Kannel W. The relationship of psychosocial factors to coronary heart disease in the Framingham Study. III. Eight-year incidence of coronary heart disease. *Am J Epidemiol* 1980; 111:37–58.

Heart: An Online Exploration. http://sln.fi.edu/biosci

Heart Information Network. http://www.heartinfo.com

Hennessy L. K., Osada J., Ordovas J. M., et al. Effects of

dietary fats and cholesterol on liver lipid content and hepatic apolipoprotein A-I, B, and E and LDL receptor mRNA levels in cebus monkeys. *J Lipid Res* 1992; 33:351–360.

Hermann W., Bierman J., and Kostner G. Comparison of effects of n-3 to n-6 fatty acids on serum level of lipoprotein(a) in patients with coronary artery disease. *Am J Cardiol* 1995; 7:459–62.

Hodis H. N. and Mack W. J. Triglyceride-rich lipoproteins and the progression of coronary artery disease. *Curr Opin Lipidol* 1995; 6:209–214.

Hodis H. N., Mack W. J., Azen S. P., et al. Triglyceride- and cholesterol-rich lipoproteins have a differential effect on mild/moderate and severe lesion progression as assessed by quantitative coronary angiography in a controlled trial of lovastatin. *Circulation* 1994; 90:42–49.

Hokanson J. E. and Austin M. A. Plasma triglyceride level is a risk factor for cardiovascular disease independent of high-density lipoprotein cholesterol levels: a meta-analysis of population-based prospective studies. *J Cardiovasc Res* 1996; 3:213–219.

Hubert H. B., Feinleib M., McNamara P. M., et al. Obesity as an independent risk factor for cardiovascular disease: A 26-year follow-up of participants in the Framingham Heart Study. *Circulation* 1983; 67:968–77.

Hulley S. B., Roseman R. H., Bawol R. D., et al. Epidemiology as a guide to clinical decisions. The association between triglyceride and coronary heart disease. *New Engl J Med* 1980; 302:1383–1389.

Hunter K., Crosbie L., Weir A., et al. The effects of structurally defined triglycerides of differing fatty acid composition on postprandial haemostasis in young, healthy men. *Atherosclerosis* 1999; 142:151–158.

International Food Information Council Foundation. http://ificinfo.health.org

Jeppesen J., Hein H., Suadicani O., et al. Triglyceride concentration and ischemic heart disease: An eight-year follow-up in the Copenhagen Male Study. *Circulation* 1998; 97:1029–1036.

Johansson J. O., Egberg N., Asplund-Carlson A., et al. Nicotinic acid treatment shifts the fibrinolytic balance favourably and decreases plasma fibrinogen in hyper-triglyceridaemic men. *J Cardiovasc Risk* 1997; 4:165–171.

Kaplan R. and Toshima M. Does a reduced fat diet cause retardation in child growth? *Prev Med* 1992, 21:33–52.

Karpe F., Steiner G., Uffelman K., et al. Postprandial lipoproteins and progression of coronary atherosclerosis. *Atherosclerosis* 1997; 106:83–97.

Kazumi T., Kawaguchi A., Hozumi T., et al. Serum HDL cholesterol values are associated with apoB-containing lipoprotein metabolism and triglyceride-body fat inter-relation in young Japanese men. *Atherosclerosis* 1997; 130:93–100.

Krauss R. M. Triglycerides and atherogenic lipoproteins: rationale for lipid management. *Am J Med* 1998; 105:58S–62S.

Kromhout D., Bosschieter E. B., and de Lezenne Coulander C. The inverse relation between fish consumption and 20-year mortality from coronary heart disease. *New Engl J Med* 1985; 312:1205–09.

Lairon D. Nutritional and metabolic aspects of postprandial lipaemia. *Reprod Nutr Dev* 1996; 36:345–355.

Lamarche B., Despres J. P., Moorjani S., et al. Prevalence of dyslipidemic phenotypes in ischemic heart disease: Prospective results from the Quebec Cardiovascular Study. *Am J Cardiol* 1995; 75:1189–1195.

Lamarche B. and Lewis G. F. Atherosclerosis prevention for the next decade: Risk assessment beyond LDL cholesterol. *Can J Cardiol* 1998; 14:841–851.

Lamarche B., Tchernof A., Dagenais G. R., et al. Small, dense LDL particles and the risk of ischemic heart disease: Prospective results from the Quebec Cardiovascular Study. *Circulation* 1997; 95:69–75.

Lamarche B., Tchernof A., Mauriege P., et al. Fasting insulin and apolipoprotein B levels and low-density lipoprotein particle size as risk factors for ischemic heart disease. *JAMA* 1998; 279:1955–1961.

LaRosa J. C., Cleary P., and Muesing R A. Effect of long-term moderate physical exercise on plasma lipoproteins. The National Exercise and Heart Disease Project. *Arch Intern Med* 1982; 142:2269–74.

Law M. R., Wald N. J., and Thompson S. G. By how much and how quickly does reduction in serum cholesterol concentration lower risk of ischaemic heart disease? *Brit Med J* 1994; 308:367–373.

Law M. R., Wald N. J., Wu T., et al. Systematic underestimations of association between serum cholesterol concentration and ischaemic heart disease in observational studies: Data from the BUPA study. *Brit Med J* 1994; 308:363–366.

Leaf A. and Weber P. C. Cardiovascular effects of n-3 fatty acids. *New Engl J Med* 1988; 318:549–57.

Levine P. H. An acute effect of cigarette smoking on platelet function: A possible link between smoking and arterial thrombosis. *Circulation* 1973; 48:619–23.

Lipid Research Clinics Program. The Lipid Research Clinics Coronary Primary Prevention Trial results. I. Reduction in incidence of coronary heart disease. *JAMA* 1984; 251:351–64.

Liu A. C., Lawn R. M., Verstuyft J. G., et al. Human apolipoprotein A-I prevents atherosclerosis associated with apolipoproteina in transgenic mice. *J Lipid Res* 1994; 35:2263–7.

Mamo J. C. L. Atherosclerosis as a postprandial disease. *Endocrinol Metab* 1995; 2:229–244.

Manninen V., Tenkanen L., Koskinen P., et al. Joint effects of serum triglyceride and LDL cholesterol and HDL cholesterol concentrations on coronary heart disease risk in the Helsinki Heart Study. Implications for treatment. *Circulation* 1992; 85:37–45.

Manzato E., Zambon A., Lapolla A., et al. Lipoprotein abnormalities in well-treated type II diabetic patients. *Diabetes Care* 1993; 16:469–75.

Mattson F. H. and Grundy S. M. Comparison of effects of dietary saturated, monounsaturated, and polyunsaturated fatty acids on plasma lipids and lipoproteins in man. *J Lipid Res* 1985; 26:194–202.

Mayo Health Oasis. http://www.mayohealth.org/mayo/common/htm/index.htm

Miek J., Dahlmans V., Princen H., et al. Effects of fenofibrate on hyperlipidemia and postprandial triglyceride metabolism in human apolipoprotein C1 transgenic mice. *Atherosclerosis* 1998; 141:77–80.

Miller M., Seidler A., Moalemi A., et al. Normal triglyceride levels and coronary artery disease events: The Baltimore Coronary Observational Long-Term Study. *J Am Coll Cardiol* 1998; 31:1252–1257.

Miller N. E. High-density lipoprotein: A major risk factor for coronary atherosclerosis. *Baillieres Clin Endocrinol Metabol* 1987; 1:603–22.

Moorjani S., Gagne C., Lupien P. J., et al. Plasma triglyceride-related decrease in high-density lipoprotein cholesterol and its association with myocardial infarction in heterozygous familial hypercholesterolaemia. *Metabolism* 1986; 35:311–316.

Must A., Jacques P. F., Dallal G. E., et al. Long-term morbidity and mortality of overweight adolescents: a follow-up of the Harvard Growth Study of 1922–1935. *N Engl J Med* 1992; 327:1350–1355.

National Cholesterol Education Program. Second report of the Expert Panel on Detection, Evaluation, and

Treatment of High Blood Cholesterol in Adults (Adult Treatment Panel II). *Circulation* 1994; 89:1333–445.

National Diabetes Data Group. Classification and diagnosis of diabetes mellitus and other categories of glucose intolerance. *Diabetes* 1979; 28:1039–57.

National Heart, Lung, and Blood Association. http://www.nhlbi.nih.gov/nhlbi/nhlbi.htm

Nicoll A., Duffield R., and Lewis B. Flux of plasma lipoproteins into human arterial intima. *Atherosclerosis* 1981; 39:229–242.

Nikkila E. A. and Aro A. Family study of serum lipids and lipoproteins in coronary heart disease. *Lancet* 1973; 1:954–959.

Nordestgaard B. G. and Zilversmit D. B. Large lipoproteins are excluded from the arterial wall in diabetic cholesterol fed rabbits. *J Lipid Res* 1988; 29:1491–1500.

Parks J. S. and Gebre A. K. Studies on the effect of dietary fish oil on the physical and chemical properties of low density lipoproteins in cynomolgus monkeys. *J Lipid Res* 1991; 32:305–15.

Patsch J. R., Miesenbock G., Hopferwieser T., et al. Relation of triglyceride metabolism and coronary artery disease: studies in the postprandial state. *Arterioscler Thromb Vasc Biol* 1992; 12:1336–1345.

Plotnick G. D., Corretti M. C., and Vogel R. A. Effect of antioxidant vitamins on the transient impairment of endothelium-dependent brachial artery vasoactivity following a single high-fat meal. *JAMA* 1997; 278:1682–1686.

Plump A. S., Scott C. J., and Breslow J. L. Human apolipoprotein A-I gene expression increases high density lipoprotein and suppresses atherosclerosis in the apolipoprotein E-deficient mouse. *Proc Natl Acad Sci USA* 1994; 91:9607–11.

Proctor S. D. and Mamo J. C. L. Arterial fatty lesions have increased uptake of chylomicron-remnants but not low density lipoprotein. *Coron Artery Dis* 1996; 7:239–245.

Proctor S. D. and Mamo J. C. L. Retention of fluorescent labelled chylomicron-remnants within the intima of the arterial wall-evidence that plaque cholesterol may be derived from postprandial lipoproteins. *Eur J Clin Invest* 1988; 28:497–503.

Ragogna F., Angeli A., Corazza S., et al. Increased J774 macrophage cytotoxicity of late postprandial triglyceride-rich lipoproteins from normolipidemic young men expressing an apolipoprotein 4 allele. *Atherosclerosis* 1997; 132:157–163.

Rapp J. H., Lespine A., Hamilton R. L., et al. Triglyceride-rich lipoproteins isolated by selected-affinity anti-apolipoprotein B immunosorption from human atherosclerotic plaque. *Arterioscler Thromb* 1994; 14:1767–74.

Roberts W. C. Atherosclerotic risk factors—are there ten or is there only one? *Am J Cardiol* 1989; 64:552–554.

Rosenberg L., Armstrong B., and Jick H. Myocardial infarction and estrogen therapy in postmenopausal women. *N Engl J Med* 1976; 294:1256–9.

Sacks F. M., Pfeffer M. A., Moye L. A., et al. The effect of pravastatin on coronary events after myocardial infarction in patients with average cholesterol levels. *New Engl J Med* 1996; 335:1001–1009.

Saito M., Eto M., and Makino I. Triglyceride-rich lipoproteins from apolipoprotein E3/2 subjects with hypertriglyceridemia enhance cholesteryl ester synthesis in human macrophages. *Atherosclerosis* 1997; 129:73–77.

Scandinavian Simvastatin Survival Study Group. Randomised trial of cholesterol lowering in 4,444 patients with coronary heart disease; the Scandinavian Survival Study. *Lancet* 1994; 344:1383–9.

Schaefer E. J., Gregg R. E., Ghiselli G., et al. Familial apolipoprotein E deficiency. *J Clin Invest* 1986; 78:1206–1219.

Schectman G., Boerboom L. E., Hannah J., et al. Dietary fish oil decreases low-density-lipoprotein clearance in nonhuman primates. *Am J Clin Nutr* 1996; 64:215–21.

Schectman G., Kaul S., and Kissebah A. Heterogeneity of low-density lipoprotein responses to fish oil concentrate in hypertriglyceridemic subjects. *Arteriosclerosis* 1989; 9:345–54.

Selby J. V., Austin M. A., Newman B., et al. LDL subclass phenotypes and the insulin resistance syndrome in women. *Circulation* 1993; 88:381–87.

Sharrett A. R., Chambless L. E., Heiss G., et al. Association of postprandial triglyceride and retinyl palmitate responses with asymptomatic carotid artery atherosclerosis in middle-aged men and women. The Atherosclerosis Risk in Communities (ARIC) Study. *Arterioscler Thromb Vasc Biol* 1995; 15:2122–9.

Shepherd J., Cobbe S. M., Ford I., et al. For the West of Scotland Coronary Prevention Study Group. Prevention of coronary heart disease with pravastatin in men with hypercholesterolaemia. *New Engl J Med* 1995; 333:1301–1307.

Simionescu N. and Simionescu M. Cellular interactions of lipoproteins with the vascular endothelium: endocytosis and transcytosis. *Targital Diagn Ther* 1991; 5:45–95.

Simons L. A. Interrelations of lipids and lipoproteins with coronary artery disease mortality in 19 countries. *Am J Cardiol* 1986; 57:5G–10G.

Simons L. A., Hickie J. B., and Balasubramaniam. On the effects of dietary n-3 fatty acids (Maxepa) on plasma lipids and lipoproteins in patients with hyperlipidemia. *Atherosclerosis* 1985; 54:75–88.

Sirtori C., Crepaldi G., Manzato E., et al. One-year treatment with ethyl esters of n-3 fatty acids in patients with hypertriglyceridemia and glucose intolerance: Reduced triglyceridemia, total cholesterol and increased HDL-C without glycemic alterations. *Atherosclerosis* 1998; 137:419–427.

Sirtori C. R. and Franceschini G. Effects of fibrates on serum lipids and atherosclerosis. *Pharmacol Ther* 1988; 37:167–91.

Sprecher D. L. Triglycerides as a risk factor for coronary artery disease. *Am J Cardiol* 1998; 82:49U–56U.

Sprecher D. L., Harris B. V., Stein E. A., et al. Higher triglycerides, lower high-density lipoprotein cholesterol, and higher systolic blood pressure in lipoprotein lipase-deficient heterozygotes: A preliminary report. *Circulation* 1996; 94:3239–3245.

Sprecher D. L., Knauer S. L., Black D. M., et al. Chylomicron-retinyl palmitate clearance in type I hyperlipidemic families. *J Clin Invest* 1991; 88:985–994.

Stacpoole P. W., Alig J., Ammon L., et al. Dose-response effects of dietary marine oil on carbohydrate and lipid metabolism in normal subjects and patients with hypertriglyceridemia. *Metabolism* 1989; 38:946–56.

Stampfer M. J., Krauss R., Ma J., et al. A prospective study of triglyceride level, low-density lipoprotein particle diameter, and risk of myocardial infarction. *JAMA* 1996; 276:822–888.

Stein E. A., Lane M., and Laskarzewski P. Comparison of statins in hypertriglyceridemia. *Am J Cardiol* 1998; 81:66B–69B.

Steiner G., Tká I., Uffelman K. D., et al. Important contribution of lipoprotein particle number to plasma triglyceride concentration in type 2 diabetes. *Atherosclerosis* 1998; 137:211–214.

Stender S. and Hjelms E. In vivo transfer of cholesterol ester from high and low density plasma lipoproteins into human aortic tissue. *Arterioscler Thromb* 1988; 8:252–262.

Takeichi S., Yukawa N., and Nakajima Y. Association of plasma triglyceride-rich lipoprotein remnants with coronary atherosclerosis in cases of sudden cardiac death. *Atherosclerosis* 1999; 142:309–315.

Tall A. R. Plasma high density lipoproteins. Metabolism and relationship to atherogenesis. *J Clin Invest* 1990; 86:379–84.

Tchernof A., Lamarche B., Nadeau A., et al. The dense LDL phenotype: Association with plasma lipoprotein levels, visceral obesity and hyperinsulinemia in men. *Diabetes Care* 1996; 19:629–637.

Thompson G. R. *A Handbook of Hyperlipidaemia.* (1990) London: Current Science.

Toft I., Bønaa K. H., Ingebretsen O. C., et al. Effects of n-3 polyunsaturated fatty acids on glucose homeostasis and blood pressure in essential hypertension. A randomized, controlled trial. *Ann Intern Med* 1995; 123: 911–8.

United States Department of Agriculture. http://www.usda.gov

Vega G. L. and Grundy S. M. Effect of statins on metabolism of apo-B-containing lipoproteins in hypertriglyceridemic men. *Am J Cardiol* 1998; 81:36B–42B.

Vogel R. A., Corretti M. C., and Plotnick G. D. Effect of a single high-fat meal on endothelial function in healthy subjects. *Am J Cardiol* 1997; 79:350–354.

Von Shacky C., Fisher S., and Weber P. C. Long-term effects of dietary marine omega-3 fatty acids upon plasma and cellular lipids, platelet function and eicosanoid formation in humans. *J Clin Invest* 1985; 76:1626–31.

Wilcox R. G., Bennett T., Brown A. M., et al. Is exercise good for high blood pressure? *Br Med J* 1982; 285:767–9.

Wilt T. J., Rubins H. B., Collins D., et al. Correlates and consequences of diffuse atherosclerosis in men with coronary heart disease. Veterans Affairs High-Density Lipoprotein Intervention Trial Study Group. *Arch Intern Med* 1996; 156:1181–8.

Witztum J. L. and Steinberg D. Role of oxidized low density lipoprotein in atherogenesis. *J Clin Investig* 1991; 88:1785–1792.

Yoshino G., Hirano T., Maeda E., et al. Effect of long-term exogenous hyperinsulinemia and fructose or glucose supplementation on triglyceride turnover in rats. *Atherosclerosis* 1997; 129:33–39.

Zilversmit D. B. Atherogenesis: A postprandial phenomenon. *Circulation* 1979; 60:473–85.

Support and Networking Resources

Cardiovascular Health Resources

American Heart Association
7272 Greenville Avenue
Dallas, TX 75231
(800) AHA-USA1
http://www.amhrt.org

Composed of physicians, scientists, and laypersons, the American Heart Association supports research, education, and community service programs aimed at reducing premature death and disability from cardiovascular disease and stroke. The AHA publishes several scholarly journals, including *Circulation*, *Circulation Research*, *Stroke*, and *Hypertension*, all of which are available in print and online. The AHA also publishes dozens of pamphlets on heart-related health issues for the consumer (see the listing on page 231).

American Society of Hypertension
515 Madison Avenue, #1515
New York, NY 10022
(212) 664-0650

The medical professional and post-graduate students who make up the American Society of Hypertension promote the development, advancement, and exchange of information on the diagnosis and treatment of hypertension. ASH publishes the *American Journal of Hypertension.*

Arizona Heart Institute Foundation
2632 N. 20th Street
Phoenix, AZ 85006
(602) 266-2200, ext. 4619
http://www.azheart.com

The Arizona Heart Institute Foundation is a nonprofit organization dedicated to preventing cardiovascular disease through research and education. The AHI provides free educational programs on health, preventive medicine, and the newest techniques for diagnosing and treating heart and blood vessel disease. The AHI also offers free brochures on many topics related to heart and blood vessel disease treatment and prevention.

Cleveland Clinic Heart Center
9500 Euclid Avenue
Cleveland, OH 44195
(216) 444-2200
(800) 223-2273, ext. 48950
http://www.ccf.org/heartcenter

The Cleveland Clinic Heart Center is one of the largest cardiovascular group practices in the world and specializes in developing new surgical interventions to treat cardiovascular diseases.

Coronary Club, Inc.
9500 Euclid Avenue, Room E4-15
Cleveland, OH 44195
(216) 444-3690

Affiliated with the Cleveland Clinic Heart Center, the
Coronary Club is comprised of doctors, patients, nurses,
therapists, educators, and other health professionals
involved in cardiac care.

Mended Hearts, Inc.
7320 Greenville Avenue
Dallas, TX 75231
http://www.mendedhearts.org

Mended Hearts is an all-volunteer organization of persons with cardiovascular disease, their family, and
friends. With more than 200 chapters, Mended Hearts
offers support to heart disease patients through its visiting
and rehabilitation programs and assistance to physicians
and other health-care workers.

National Heart, Lung, and Blood Institute
31 Center Drive, MSC 2480
Bethesda, MD 20892
(301) 496-4236
http://www.nhlbi.nih.gov/nhlbi/nhlbi.htm

The National Heart, Lung, and Blood Institute supports and conducts research, clinical investigations and
trials, observational studies, and demonstration and education programs that concern diseases of the heart, lungs,
blood, and blood vessels.

National Hypertension Association
324 E. 30th Street
New York, NY 10016
(212) 889-3557

The National Hypertension Association is composed of physicians, medical researchers, and business professionals who seek to prevent the complications of hypertension. The NHA conducts programs to educate physicians and the public; research into the causes of hypertension; and conducts hypertension and hypercholesterol detection programs.

National Stroke Association
96 Iverness Drive East, Suite 1
Englewood, CO 80112
(303) 649-9299
(800) STROKES
http://www.stroke.org

The National Stroke Association seeks to reduce the incidence and impact of stroke by changing the way stroke is viewed and treated. The NSA offers public and patient education, professional education, and support to stroke survivors and their families through counseling and referrals to NSA chapters and support groups. It also conducts research. The NSA sponsors the scholarly *Journal of Stroke and Cerebrovascular Diseases*.

Nutrition Resources

American Dietetic Association
216 W. Jackson Boulevard
Chicago, IL 60606
(312) 899-0040
(800) 366-1655
http://www.eatright.org

A group of dietetic professionals and registered dieti-
cians, the American Dietetic Association serves the public by promoting optimal nutrition and health. The ADA
seeks to positively influence the nutritional status of the
food served to the public in hospitals, schools, colleges
and universities, business, and industry. The ADA also
publishes the scholarly *Journal of the American Dietetic
Association.*

American Society for Nutritional Services
9650 Rockville Pike
Bethesda, MD 20814-3990
(301) 530-7050
http://www.faseb.org/asan

The American Society of Nutritional Services is a
research society dedicated to improving the public's quality of life through the science of nutrition. The ASNS
conducts research, fosters educational and training in
nutrition, upholds the standard of ethics in research, and
provides a forum for the discussion and dissemination of
nutrition research results through its publication, the
Journal of Nutrition.

Food and Drug Administration
5600 Fisher's Lane
Rockville, MD 20857
(301) 827-2410
http://www.fda.gov

The U.S. Food and Drug Administration, a division of the Department of Health and Human Services, is responsible for protecting American consumers by enforcing the Federal Food, Drug, and Cosmetic Act and several related public health laws written to ensure the safety of the food we eat, cosmetics we use, medicines we take, and the medical and radiation-emitting devices (such as microwaves) we use.

International Food Information Council Foundation
1100 Connecticut Avenue N.W. Suite 430
Washington, DC, 20036
http://wifcinfo.heatlh.org

The International Food Information Council is a nonprofit organization that provides scientific information on food safety and nutrition to journalists, health professionals, educators, government officials, and the general public.

Society for Nutrition Education
2850 Metro Drive, Suite 416
Minneapolis, MN 55425
(612) 854-0035

The Society for Nutrition Education conducts and promotes nutrition education research and disseminates scientifically based food and nutrition information to promote the nutritional well-being of the public. The Society's activities include conducting food and nutrition education programs for the public as well as professionals, research, skills development for professionals, and legislation and public policy.

United States Department of Agriculture
Food and Nutrition Service
14th Street and Independence Avenue SW, Room 240-E
Washington, DC 20250
(202) 720-7711
http://www.usda.gov/fcs/fcs.htm

Formerly known as the Food and Consumer Service, the Food and Nutrition Service administers the nutrition assistance program (Food Stamp Program, National School Lunch Program, etc.) of the U.S. Department of Agriculture. Through these and other programs, the Food and Nutrition Service seeks to provide low-income families with better access to nutritious food.

Diabetes Resources

American Diabetes Association
1660 Duke Street
Alexandria, VA 22314
(800) DIABETES
http://www.diabetes.org

With offices in more than 800 communities, the American Diabetes Association is the nation's leading nonprofit health organization in the field of diabetes. The ADA strives to prevent and cure diabetes and to improve the quality of life of people who have the disease. The ADA funds research, publishes scientific findings, and provides information and other services to people with diabetes, their families, healthcare professionals, and the public. The ADA publishes the consumer-oriented *Diabetes Forecast* as well as several professional-level journals

National Diabetes Information Clearinghouse
1 Information Way
Bethesda, MD 20892-3560
(301) 654-3327
http://www.niddk.nih.gov/health/diabetes/ndic.htm

The National Diabetes Information Clearinghouse, a part of the National Institute of Diabetes and Digestive and Kidney Diseases, which is part of the National Institutes of Health, offers publications, both in print and online, to educate consumers about diabetes. The NIDDK also maintains an online database of books, articles, audiovisual materials, and more.

General Medical Resources

American Academy of Family Physicians
8880 Ward Parkway
Kansas City, MO 64114-2797
(816) 333-9700
http://www.aafp.org

The American Academy of Family Physicians is a national, nonprofit medical association that promotes and maintains standards for family doctors.

American Medical Association
515 North State Street
Chicago, IL 60610
(312) 464-4818
http://www.ama-assn.org

The American Medical Association is the leading voice of the American medical profession. To carry out is mission "to promote the art and science of medicine and the betterment of public health," the AMA provides the latest medical information to members and the public through the *Journal of the American Medical Association*, helps educate programs, provides physician placement service and counseling on practice management, and represents the medical profession before Congress. The AMA also offers physician and hospital-locating services.

Public Health Resources

Centers for Disease Control and Prevention
1600 Clifton Road NE
Atlanta, GA 30333
(404) 639-3311
http://www.cdc.gov

A division of the Department of Health and Human Services, the Centers for Disease Control and Prevention is a collection of institutes and offices dedicated to promoting health and quality of life by preventing and controlling disease, injury, and disability.

National Health Information Center
U.S. Department of Health and Human Services
P.O. Box 1133
Washington, DC 20013
(301) 565-4167
(800) 336-4797
http://www.nhic-nt.health.org

The National Health Information Center is a health information referral service that connects health professionals and consumers who have health questions to organizations that can provide answers to their questions. The Health Information Resource Database includes more than 1,000 organizations and government offices that provide health information upon request. Entries include contact information, abstracts, and information about publications and services the organizations provide.

National Institutes of Health
Building 1, Room B156
1 Center Drive MSC0122
Bethesda, MD 20892-0148
(301) 496-1461
http://www.nih.gov

Comprised of 24 separate institutes, centers, and divisions, the National Institutes of Health is another division of the Department of Health and Human Services, whose mission is to uncover medical knowledge that will lead to the betterment of the public health. Toward this goal, the NIH supports the research of scientists throughout the country and abroad in addition to conducting its own research.

World Health Organization
Regional Office for the Americas
Pan American Health Organization
525 23rd Street NW
Washington, DC 20037
(202) 974-3000
http://www.who.org

The objective of WHO is the attainment by people worldwide of the highest possible level of physical, emotional, and social health. Among WHO's many functions are to stimulate work on the prevention and control of epidemic, endemic, and other diseases; to promote the improvement of nutrition, housing, sanitation, recreation, economic and working conditions, and other aspects of environmental hygiene; to promote improved standards of teaching and training in the health, medical, and related professions; to establish international standards for biological and pharmaceutical products; and to standardize diagnostic procedures.

Complementary and Alternative Medicine Resources

National Center for Complementary and Alternative Medicine
P.O. Box 8218
Silver Spring, Maryland 20907-8218
(888) 644-6226
http://altmed.od.nih.gov/nccam

A division of the National Institutes of Health, the National Center for Complementary and Alternative Medicine facilities and conducts research and training and disseminates information on complementary and alternative medicine to medical professionals and the public.

Quackwatch
http://www.quackwatch.com

Quackwatch, Inc. is a nonprofit corporation whose purpose is to combat health-related fallacies and frauds and consumer gullibility. The Quackwatch Web site contains numerous and lengthy articles and reports about complementary and alternative medical practices from herbal remedies to chelation therapy.

Women's Health Resources

American Medical Women's Association
801 North Fairfax Street, Suite 400
Alexandria, VA 22314
(703) 383-0500
http://www.amwa-doc.org/index.html

The American Medical Women's Association is a national organization of women physicians and medical students dedicated to promoting women's health and increasing the influence of women in all aspects of the medical profession. The AMWA publishes educational materials regarding women's health for the public and conducts educational programs for women physicians.

National Women's Health Network
514 10th Street NW, Suite 400
Washington, DC 20004
(202) 344-1140
http://www.aoa.dhhs.gov/aoa/dir/203.html

A cooperative effort of the National Institute on Aging and the Administration on Aging, the National Women's Health Network's mission is to ensure that women have access to quality, affordable health care. The NWHN also serves as a national clearinghouse for information on women's health issues and distributes educational materials to the public.

National Women's Health Resource Center
120 Albany Street, Suite 820
New Brunswick, NJ 08901
(877) 986-9472
http://www.healthywomen.org

Tha National Women's Health Resource Center seeks to educate consumers about women's health through newsletters (including its own *National Women's Health Report*), health databases, health Web sites, and NWHRC national partners. For a fee, the NWHRC will perform research in response to specific health concerns.

Senior Health Resources

Administration on Aging
330 Independence Avenue SW
Washington, DC 20201
(202) 619-0724
(800) 677-1116
http://www.aoa.gov

A division of the Department of Health and Human Services, the Administration on Aging is the federal advocate agency for older Americans. The goal of the AOA is to heighten awareness among other federal agencies, organizations, and the public about the contributions that older Americans make to the country and alert them to the needs of older people. Furthermore, the AOA seeks to empower older people and their caregivers by making them aware of the benefits and services available to them.

American Association of Retired Persons
601 E Street, NW
Washington, DC 20049
(202) 434-AARP
http://www.aarp.org

The American Association of Retired Persons is the nation's leading organization for people age 50 and older. With a network of chapters throughout the country, AARP advocates the interests of those aged 50 and older through dedication, lobbying, and community services.

National Institute on Aging
P.O. Box 8057
Gaithersburg, MD 20898
(800) 222-2225
http://www.nih.gov/nia

The National Institute on Aging is one of the National Institutes of Health. The NIA promotes healthy aging by conducting and supporting biomedical, social, and behavioral research and also produces science-based educational materials for the general public on topics related to health and aging.

Medical Resource Sites on the Internet

Although many of the organizations listed above have Web sites, the Web sites that you'll find below have been singled out for their breadth of scope. On these sites you'll find information on every health topic under the sun, not just one particular facet of health.

This list is not intended to be comprehensive—for, unlike books, the Web is a dynamic medium in which new sites suddenly appear while old ones vanish—but is merely intended as a springboard, a helpful first step, for you to locate the health information you desire.

healthfinder
http://www.healthfinder.org/default.htm

healthfinder is a consumer health and human services information Web site developed by the U.S. Department of Health and Human Services. healthfinder has links to all sorts of health Web sites, including government agencies, nonprofit organizations, online publications, databases, and support groups.

Healthtouch
http://www.healthtouch.com

Maintained by Medical Strategies, Inc., a designer, developer, and manufacturer of custom interactive multimedia systems and software, Healthtouch is a collection of health databases. The Drug Information Database contains information on prescription and over-the-counter medications, such as common drug uses, proper use of medications, and potential drug side effects. In the Health Information Database you will find information on an array of health topics, from family planning to diet and nutrition. All of the information found on Healthtouch comes from established government and academic institutions and corporations.

Intelihealth
http://www.intelihealth.com

Intelihealth is a multimedia company that is a cooperative effort between Aetna U.S. Healthcare and Johns Hopkins University. Medical news is updated daily and special features include "Ask the Doc," in which a Johns Hopkins doctor will respond to your health questions, the answers for which will be posted on the site, and a free health e-mail service wherein Johns Hopkins will notify you of any news in a health topic of your choiee.

Mayo Health Oasis
http://www.mayohealth.org/mayo/common/htm/index.htm

Mayo Health Oasis is the Web site of the Mayo Clinic. The site is divided into various centers, including those dealing with cancer, nutrition, and men's women's and children's health. In addition, there is an alternative medicine index and the site if fully searchable.

Medscape
http://www.medscape.com

Owned and operated by Medscape, Inc., Medscape gathers information from medical journals, medical news providers, medical education programs, and material created expressly for Medscape. The site is organized as a set of file folders that includes "Specialties"—for current and archived articles organized by medical specialty or clinical topic "News"—for the latest medical news from a variety of national and international sources; "Library"—which contains a drug search resource and medical dictionary; and several more.

New York Online Access to Health (NOAH)
http://www.noah.cuny.edu

New York Online Access to Health is the product of a partnership between the City University of New York, the

Metropolitan New York Library Council, the New York Academy of Medicine, and the New York Public Library. NOAH is a bilingual (English and Spanish) health information site.

National Library of Medicine
http://www.nlm.niv.gov

   Maintained by the National Institutes of Health, the National Library of Medicine is the world's largest biomedical library. The National Library of Medicine contains 40 online databases, foremost among them Medline, a bibliographic database covering the fields of medicine, nursing, dentistry, veterinary medicine, the health-care system, and the preclinical sciences. Medline contains bibliographic citations and author abstracts from over 3,900 biomedical journals published in the United States and 70 foreign countries during the past four years (older articles are indexed in companion databases, e.g., MED93, MED90, etc).

Books

365 Ways to Get Out the Fat
American Heart Association, Times Books, 1998.

American Diabetes Association Complete Guide to Diabetes
American Diabetes Association, 1997.

The American Diabetes Association Guide to Healthy Restaurant Eating
Hope S. Warshaw, American Diabetes Association, 1998.

The American Dietetic Association's Complete Food and Nutrition Guide
Roberta Larson Duyff, Chronimed, 1996.

American Heart Association Family Guide to Stroke Treatment, Recovery and Prevention
American Heart Association, Times Books, 1996.

American Heart Association Fitting in Fitness: Hundreds of Simple Ways to Put More Physical Activity into Your Life
American Heart Association, Times Books, 1997.

American Heart Association Guide to Heart Attack Treatment, Recovery, and Prevention
American Heart Association, Times Books, 1998.

American Heart Association's Your Heart: An Owner's Manual
American Heart Association, Times Books, 1995.

An Emotionally Normal Heart Attack
Richard Tenney, Nova Science, 1998.

Brand Name Fat and Cholesterol Counter
American Heart Association, Times Books, 1995.

Cholesterol: Your Guide to a Healthy Heart
Neil J. Stone (Editor) et al., NAL/Dutton, 1993.

The Cholesterol Counter
Annette B. Natow and Jo-Ann Heslin, Pocket Books, 1998.

Cut the Fat!
American Dietetic Association, HarperCollins, 1996.

Dr. Dean Ornish's Program for Reversing Heart Disease: The Only System Scientifically Proven to Reverse Heart Disease Without Drugs or Surgery
Dean Ornish, Ballantine Books, 1996.

Diabetes A to Z: What You Need to Know About Diabetes—Simply Put
American Diabetes Association, 1998.

Eating Smart: The ABCs of the New Food Literacy
Jeanne Jones, Macmillan, 1994.

The Eight-week Cholesterol Cure: How to Lower Your Blood Cholesterol By Up to 40% Without Drugs or Deprivation
Robert E. Kowalski and Albert A. Kattus, HarperCollins, 1990.

Every Person's Guide to Antioxidants
John R. Smythies, Rutgers University Press, 1998.

The Female Heart: The Truth About Women and Heart Disease
Marianne J. Legato and Carol Colman, Prentice Hall, 1991.

Fighting the Silent Killer: How Men and Women Can Prevent and Cope with Heart Disease Today
Peter F. Cohn, and Joan K. Cohn, A.K. Peters Ltd., 1993.

From Hypertension to Heart Failure
M. Bohm and John H. Laragh (Editors), Springer-Verlag, 1998.

Good Cholesterol, Bad Cholesterol
Eli M. Roth and Sandra L. Streicher, Prima Publishing, 1995.

Good Fat, Bad Fat: How to Lower Your Cholesterol and Reduce the Odds of a Heart Attack
William P. Castelli and Glen C. Griffin, Fisher Books, 1997.

Heal Your Heart: How You Can Prevent or Reverse Heart Disease
K. Lance Gould, Rutgers University Press, 1998.

Healthy Heart Handbook: How to Prevent and Reverse Heart Disease, Lower Your Risk of Heart Attack and Cancer, Reduce Stress, Lose Weight Without Hunger
Neal Pinckney, Health Communications, 1996.

The Healthy Heart Walking Book: The American Heart Association Walking Program
The American Heart Association, 1995.

The Heart Attack Prevention and Recovery Handbook
Jack Gillis, Hartley and Marks Publishers, 1997.

Heart-Aches: Heart Disease and the Psychology of the Broken Heart
Rudiger Dahlke, Bluestar Communication Corp., 1996.

The Heart Disease Sourcebook
Roger Cicala, Lowell House, 1997.

Heart Fitness for Life: The Essential Guide to Preventing and Reversing Heart Disease
Mary P. McGowan and Jo McGowan Chopra, Oxford University Press, 1997.

Johns Hopkins Complete Guide to Preventing and Reversing Heart Disease
Peter O. Kwiterovich Jr., Prima Publishing, 1998.

Lady Killer: Heart Disease: Women at Risk
Suzanne Cambre, Pritchett and Hall, 1995.

Living Well, Staying Well: The Ultimate Guide to Help Prevent Heart Disease and Cancer
American Heart Association and the American Cancer Society, Times Books, 1999.

The McDougall Program for a Healthy Heart: A Life-Saving Approach to Preventing and Treating Heart Disease
Mary McDougall and John A McDougall, Plume, 1998.

Nutrition for the Prime of Life: The Adult Guide to Healthier Living
Hugh J. McDonald and Frances Sapone, Plenum Press, 1993.

The Official Pocket Guide to Diabetic Exchanges
American Dietetic Association, 1998.

Reversing Heart Disease
Julian M. Whitaker, Warner Books, 1995.

Skim the Fat: A Practical and Up-to-Date Food Guide
American Dietetic Association, Chronimed, 1995.

Trans Fatty Acids and Coronary Heart Disease Risk
P. M. Kris-Etherton et al., International Life Sciences Institute, 1995.

Winning with Heart Attack: A Complete Program for Health and Well-Being
Harris H. McIlwain (Editor) et al., Prometheus Books, 1994.

Women and Heart Disease
Edward B. Diethrich and Carol Cohan, Ballantine Books, Inc., 1994.

The Women's Concise Guide to a Healthier Heart
Stephanie A. Eisenstate, et al., Harvard University Press,
    1997.

Your Heart: Questions You Have . . . Answers you Need
People's Medical Society, 1996.

Your Personal Nutritionist: Antioxidant Counter
Edward R. Blonz et al., Signet, 1996.

Cookbooks

*American Heart Association Around the World Cook-
    book: Healthy Recipes with International Flavor*
American Heart Association, Times Books, 1996.

*American Heart Association Low-Fat, Low-Cholesterol
    Cookbook: Healthy Easy to Make Recipes That Taste
    Great*
Times Books, 1995

*American Heart Association Low-Salt Cookbook: A
    Complete Guide to Reducing Sodium and Fat in the
    Diet*
Rodman D. Starke and Mary Winston (Editors), Times
    Books, 1990.

*American Heart Association Quick and Easy Cookbook:
    More Than 200 Delicious, Heart-Healthful Recipes for
    the Whole Family*
Times Books, 1998.

*Arizona Heart Institute Foundation Cookbook: A Renais-
    sance in Good Eating*
Arizona Heart Institute Foundation, 1993.

Cooking à la Heart
Linda Hachfield, Betsy Eykyn, and Mankato Heart
   Health Program Foundation, Appletree Press, 1992.

Don't Eat Your Heart Out Cookbook
Joseph C. Piscatella, Workman Publishing Co., 1994.

The Healthy Heart Cookbook
Lisa A. Hooper and Lisa Hooper Talley (Editors),
   Oxmoor House, 1992.

Heart Smart Cookbook
Wichita Eagle and Beacon Publishing Co. Inc., 1996.

The Heart Smart Healthy Exchanges Cookbook
Joanna M. Lund, Perigree, 1999.

The Love Your Heart Low Cholesterol Cookbook
Surrey Books, 1993.

The New American Heart Association Cookbook
American Heart Association, Times Books, 1999.

*Newstart Lifestyle Cookbook: More than 200 Heart-
   Healthy Recipes Featuring Whole Plant Foods*
Weimar Institute, Sally J. Christenson, and Frances De
   Vries, Thomas Nelson, 1997.

*Stanford University Healthy Heart Cookbook and Life
   Plan: Over 200 Delicious Low-fat Recipes Plus the
   Revolutionary 25 Gram Plan from the World-
   Renouned Medical Center*
John Speer Schroeder et al., Chronicle Books, 1997.

Vegetarian Homestyle Cooking
J. Tiberio and S. Massaglia, Appletree, 1998.

The Wellness Lowfat Cookbook: Hundreds of Delicious Recipes and a Revolutionary New Eating Plan That Can Help Prevent Heart Disease
University of California and the Wellness Cooking School (Editors), Random House, 1994.

Newsletters

The Cleveland Clinic Heart Advisor
P.O. Box 420235
Palm Coast, FL 32142-0235
(800) 829-2506

Consumer Reports on Health
Box 56356
Boulder, CO 80322
(800) 234-2188

Environmental Nutrition
P.O. Box 420235
Palm Coast, FL 32142
(800) 829-5384

FDA Consumer
Superintendent of Documents
Government Printing Office
Washington, DC 20402
(202) 512-1800

Harvard Health Letter
P.O. Box 420300
Palm Coast, FL 32142
(800) 829-9045
http://www.harvardhealthpubs.org

The Johns Hopkins Health Insider
97 Commerce Way
P.O. Box 7029
Dover, DE 19903
(800) 988-1127
http://www.jhinsider.com

Mayo Clinic Health Letter
Subscription Services
P.O. Box 53889
Boulder, CO 80322
(800) 333-9037

Tufts University Health and Nutrition Letter
P.O. Box 57857
Boulder, CO 80322
(800) 274-7581

University of California at Berkeley Wellness Letter
Health Letter Associates
P.O. Box 420235
Palm Coast, FL 32142
(800) 829-9080

Audio Tapes

*The Healthy Heart Walking Workouts for a Lifetime of
   Fitness*
American Heart Association, 1995.

American Heart Association Brochures

American Heart Association offers a number of educational
brochures on a variety of heart health topics, from surgery

to nutrition. You can order up to ten brochures at no cost by calling (800) AHA-USA1. A sampling is listed below.

About High Blood Pressure
This pamphlet explains what high blood pressure is and how it affects your body, risk factors that are within and beyond your control, and the range of treatments available.

American Heart Association Diet: An Eating Plan for Healthy Americans
This pamphlet presents a dietary plan for Americans over the age of two to help them reduce saturated fat, total fat, cholesterol, and sodium in their diet in order to control blood cholesterol and blood pressure.

Cholesterol and Your Heart
A fat and cholesterol content chart for popular foods is included in this pamphlet.

Dietary Treatment of Hypercholesterolemia (for Patients)
Written for patients with hypercholesterolemia, this booklet incorporates professional dietary counseling as part of a program to reduce cholesterol.

Heart Attack
This brochure explains the connection between heart attack, angina pectoris, and coronary atherosclerosis and tells you what to do in case of a heart attack.

Heart Attack and Stroke Signals and Action
Cardiovascular and cerebrovascular disease are among the leading causes of death in the United States. This brochure discusses the scope and impact of these

killers and tells how to recognize and respond to heart attack and stroke.

How to Have Your Cake and Eat It Too
This pamphlet offers hints on how to reduce serum cholesterol by reducing cholesterol and saturated fat. It also includes a chart that lists the fat, saturated fat, and cholesterol contents of foods commonly eaten by Americans.

How to Read Food Labels
The AHA created this pamphlet in response to the new FDA food label. It provides basic information for use by consumers, dietitians, and health educators.

How You Can Help Your Doctor Treat Your High Blood Pressure
This brochure focuses on drugs used to treat high blood pressure and their common side effects.

Just Move
As exercise is integral for a healthy heart, this leaflet depicts the types of exercise which might be recommended to promote cardiovascular fitness. It lists several factors one should consider before starting an exercise program and explains how to exercise.

Nutritious Nibbles: A Guide to Healthy Snacking
Recognizing that snacking is a part of most Americans' lives, this brochure offers tips on how to snack healthfully. Included are recipes suggestions and a list of healthy and unhealthy snack choices.

Smoking and Heart Disease
Everyone knows that cigarette smoking can lead to

lung cancer. However, this pamphlet describes the relationship between cigarette smoking and cardio-vascular diseases, including atherosclerosis, heart attack, peripheral vascular disease, and angina pec-toris.

Tips for Eating Out

Eating out can wreak havoc on a diet. This brochure shows you how to eat out healthfully by giving you general guidelines and questions to ask wait staff when ordering food.

What Every Woman Should Know About High Blood Pressure

Women experience high blood pressure too. This pam-phlet discusses the latest findings on high blood pres-sure and women. Also covered is the relationship between high blood pressure and oral contraceptives, pregnancy, menopause, and the predisposition to high blood pressure in African American women.

What to Ask About High Blood Pressure

Many people are intimidated by doctors and doctors' offices and don't know what questions to ask. This pamphlet tells you what questions to ask your doctor about high blood pressure, lifestyle changes you may have to make, and medications that you may take.

What You Should Know About Stroke

This pamphlet describes the various types of stroke, their warning signs, risk factors, treatment, and rehabilita-tion.

Index

Complete and Authoritative
Health Care Books From Wholecare

THE ARTHRITIS SOLUTION
80778-5/$5.99 US/$7.99 Can   by Robert G. Lahita, M.D., Ph.D.

WHAT DOCTORS DON'T TELL YOU:
**The Truth About the Dangers
of Modern Medicine**   by Lynne McTaggart
80761-0/$6.99 US/$8.99 Can

LIVING WELL WITH LACTOSE INTOLERANCE
80642-8/$5.99 US/$7.99 Can   by Jaime Aranda-Michel, M.D.
and Donald S. Vaughan

MAKE YOUR MEDICINE SAFE
**How to Prevent Side Effects
from the Drugs You Take**   by Jay Sylvan Cohen, M.D.
79075-0/$7.50 US/$9.50 Can

THE OSTEOPOROSIS CURE
**Reverse the Crippling Effects
with New Treatments**   by Harris McIlwain, M.D.
79336-9/$5.99 US/$7.99 Can   and Debra Fulghum Bruce

MIGRANES: Everything You Need to Know About
Their Cause and Cure
79077-7/$5.99 US/$7.99 Can   by Arthur Elkind, M.D.

Alternative Healing Approaches

MSM: THE NATURAL PAIN RELIEF REMEDY
by Deborah Mitchell
80899-4/$5.99 US/$7.99 Can

KAVA
NATURE'S STRESS RELIEF
by Kathryn M. Connor, M.D. and Donald S. Vaughan
80641-X/$5.99 US/$7.99 Can

ST. JOHN'S WORT
NATURE'S MOOD BOOSTER
Everything You Need to Know about This
Natural Antidepressant
by Michael E. Thase, M.D. and Elizabeth E. Loredo
80288-0/$5.99 US/$7.99 Can

GINKGO
NATURE'S BRAIN BOOSTER
by Alan H. Pressman, D.C., Ph.D., C.C.N.
with Helen Tracy
80640-1/$5.99 US/$7.99 Can

A HANDBOOK OF NATURAL FOLK REMEDIES
by Elena Oumano, Ph.D.
78448-3/$5.99 US/$7.99 Can